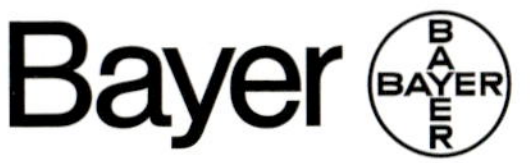

Jo Ellen Schweinle, MD
Director
Scientific Relations

AF330087

Dear Doctor:

We are pleased to present you with Dr. Stuart Howards' *Review of Adult and Pediatric Urology*, a companion to the third edition of Gillenwater et al's classic text.

The Bayer Corporation, Pharmaceutical Division, maker of Cipro® (ciprofloxacin HCl) Tablets and Cipro® I.V. (ciprofloxacin), hopes that you will find this a useful reference work.

We understand that this book has proven particularly helpful for urology residents preparing for the boards and for practicing urologists seeking recertification. Whatever your current certification status, we are confident that this review will prove a valuable addition to your reference library.

Cordially,

Schweinle, M. D.

Jo Ellen Schweinle, MD
Director, Scientific Relations

Compliments of Bayer Corporation,
Pharmaceutical Division

Maker of

Cipro® I.V. (ciprofloxacin)
Cipro® (ciprofloxacin HCl) Tablets

REVIEW OF

the Third Edition of

Adult and Pediatric Urology

Stuart S. Howards

Mosby

St. Louis Baltimore Boston Carlsbad Chicago Naples New York
Philadelphia Portland London Madrid Mexico City Singapore
Sydney Tokyo Toronto Wiesbaden

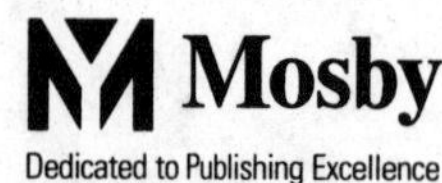**Mosby**

Dedicated to Publishing Excellence

A Times Mirror Company

Publisher: Anne S. Patterson
Editor: Susie H. Baxter
Editorial Assistant: Christy R. Stewart
Project Manager: Gayle May Morris
Typographer: Diana J. Thomson
Manufacturing Supervisor: Betty Richmond
Cover Designer: Kay Kramer

Printed in the United States of America

Mosby-Year Book, Inc.
11830 Westline Industrial Drive
St. Louis, Missouri 64146

International Standard Book Number
0-8151-4713-9

96 97 98 99 00 / 9 8 7 6 5 4 3 2 1

Preface

Review of the Third Edition of Adult and Pediatric Urology has been written to complement the third edition of Adult and Pediatric Urology. This book is intended to test the knowledge of residents preparing for exams, which may require more study, practicing urologists seeking recertification and urologists in general. It can be used to identify areas of weakness as well as areas that are well understood by the reader. It may also serve as an interesting method of enhancing the relevant information base of any urologist. Questions are drawn from each chapter in the textbook and consist of both basic science and clinically relevant topics. To simulate standardized testing format, each question is multiple choice. We have asked each contributor to state the questions clearly and provide five possible answers, along with rationale to briefly explain to the reader why the answer is correct. To aid in further understanding, each correct answer is referenced to a specific page in the textbook where the topic is discussed in detail.

I would like to thank the authors who contributed questions and answers in such a short time frame so that this book would be available alongside the textbook. I would also like to express my gratitude to my assistant, Carol Chowdhry, and to Christy Stewart at Mosby-Year Book, for their patience and diligence in keeping everything on track.

Stuart S. Howards

CONTRIBUTORS

Vaseem Ali, M.D.
Division of Urology
The University of Texas Medical School
Houston, Texas

Richard J. Andrassy, M.D.
Professor of Surgery and Pediatrics
Chief, Division of Pediatric Surgery
Department of Surgery
University of Texas Medical School
Houston, Texas

David M. Barrett, M.D.
Professor and Chair
Department of Urology
Mayo Clinic
Rochester, Minnesota

Laurence S. Baskin, M.D.
Assistant Professor of Pediatrics
  and Urology
Department of Urology
University of California
  School of Medicine
San Francisco, California

Mark F. Bellinger, M.D.
Associate Professor
Division of Urology
University of Pittsburgh
  School of Medicine
Director, Department of Pediatric
  Urology
Children's Hospital of Pittsburgh
Pittsburgh, Pennsylvania

George S. Benson, M.D.
Professor
Division of Urology
University of Texas Medical School
Houston, Texas

David Bloom, M.D.
Professor
Department of Surgery
Section of Urology
Chief of Pediatric Urology
University of Michigan
  School of Medicine
Ann Arbor, Michigan

Bruce Blyth, M.D.
Clinical Assistant Professor
Department of Surgery
University of Colorado Health
  Sciences Center
Denver, Colorado

Michel A. Boileau, M.D.
Bend Urology Associates
St. Charles Medical Center
Bend, Oregon

Wade Bushman, M.D., Ph.D.
Assistant Professor
Department of Urology
Northwestern University Medical School
Chicago, Illinois

Douglas A. Canning, M.D.
Assistant Professor of Urology
Department of Surgery
University of Pennsylvania
  School of Medicine
Philadelphia, Pennsylvania

William J. Catalona, M.D.
Professor and Chief
Division of Urologic Surgery
Washington University
  School of Medicine
St. Louis, Missouri

Marc Cendron, M.D.
Section of Urology
Dartmouth-Hitchcock Medical Center
Lebannon, New Hampshire

Mark Chazen, M.D.
Department of Urology
State University of New York
  at Buffalo
School of Medicine and Biomedical
  Sciences
Buffalo, New York

Peter L. Choyke, M.D.
Professor
Department of Radiology
Uniformed Services University of
  the Health Sciences
Chief, MRI
Henry M. Jackson Foundation at the
  Clinical Center
Bethesda, Maryland

Ralph V. Clayman, M.D.
Professor of Urology and Radiology
Departments of Surgery (Urology)
  and Radiology
Washington University
  School of Medicine
St. Louis, Missouri

Bo L.R.A. Coolsaet, M.D.
Professor of Urology
State University of Utrecht
Utrecht, The Netherlands

Douglas E. Coplen, M.D.
Assistant Professor
Division of Urologic Surgery
Washington University
  School of Medicine
St. Louis, Missouri

Joseph N. Corriere, Jr., M.D.
Professor of Surgery
Division of Urology
University of Texas Medical School
Houston, Texas

Barbara Y. Croft, Ph.D.
Associate Professor
Department of Radiology
University of Virginia
  Health Sciences Center
Charlottesville, Virginia

William C. DeWolf, M.D.
Urologist-in-Chief
Urologic Oncology
Director, Urology Research Laboratories
Beth Israel Hospital
Boston, Massachusetts

John P. Donohue, M.D.
Distinguished Professor and Chairman
Indiana University School of Medicine
Indianapolis, Indiana

John W. Duckett, M.D.
Professor
Department of Urology
University of Pennsylvania
  School of Medicine;
Director, Pediatric Urology
Children's Hospital of Philadelphia
Philadelphia, Pennsylvania

Richard F. Edlich, M.D., Ph.D.
Distinguished Professor of Plastic
  Surgery and Biomedical Engineering
Department of Plastic Surgery
University of Virginia Health
  Sciences Center
Charlottesville, Virginia

Gary J. Faerber, M.D.
Assistant Professor
Section of Urology
University of Michigan
  School of Medicine
Ann Arbor, Michigan

R. Sherburne Figenshau, M.D.
Division of Urology
Washington University
  School of Medicine
St. Louis, Missouri

Loulie M. Fisher, M.D.
Private Practice
Pensacola, Florida

Stuart M. Flechner, M.D.
Department of Urology
Cleveland Clinic Foundation
Cleveland, Ohio

Richard S. Foster, M.D.
Associate Professor
Department of Urology
Indiana University School of Medicine
Indianapolis, Indiana

Jackson E. Fowler, Jr., M.D.
Professor of Surgery and Chief
Division of Urology
University of Mississippi
  School of Medicine
Jackson, Mississippi

Jay Y. Gillenwater, M.D.
Hovey S. Dabney Professor
Department of Urology
University of Virginia
  Health Sciences Center
Charlottesville, Virginia

John T. Grayhack, M.D.
Professor
Department of Urology
Northwestern University Medical School
Chicago, Illinois

Marko Gudziak, M.D.
Division of Urology
The University of Texas Medical School
Houston, Texas

M. Craig Hall, M.D.
Department of Urology
The University of Texas
MD Anderson Cancer Center
Houston, Texas

Faruk Hadziselimovic, M.D.
Director
Institute of Andrology
Listal, Switzerland

Terry W. Hensle, M.D.
Professor
Department of Urology
Columbia University College of
  Physicians and Surgeons
Director of Pediatric Urology
Babies Hospital-Columbia
  Presbyterian Medical Center
New York, New York

Ernest E. Hodge, M.D.
Department of Urology
Cleveland Clinic Foundation
Cleveland, Ohio

Stuart S. Howards, M.D.
Professor
Department of Urology
University of Virginia
  Health Sciences Center
Charlottesville, Virginia

M'Liss A. Hudson, M.D.
Assistant Professor
Division of Urologic Surgery
Washington University
  School of Medicine
St. Louis, Missouri

Dale Huff, M.D.
Professor of Pathology
University of Pittsburgh
  School of Medicine
Director
Developmental Perinatal Pathology
Magee-Womens Hospital
Pittsburgh, Pennsylvania

Alan D. Jenkins, M.D.
Associate Professor
Department of Urology
University of Virginia
  Health Sciences Center
Charlottesville, Virginia

Scott B. Jennings, M.D.
Fellow in Urologic Oncology
Surgery Branch, National Cancer Institute
Bethesda, Maryland

Judith M. Joyce, M.D.
Associate Director
Nuclear Medicine
The Western Pennsylvania Hospital
Director
Nuclear Medicine
Suburban General Hospital
Pittsburgh, Pennsylvania

Panayotis P. Kelalis, M.D.
Anson L. Clark Professor of
  Pediatric Urology
Chairman, Department of Urology
Mayo Clinic and Mayo Foundation
Rochester, Minnesota

Charles D. Kellum, M.D.
Department of Radiology
HCA Colliseum Park Hospital
Macon, Georgia

Stephen A. Koff, M.D.
Professor of Surgery
Division of Urology
Ohio State University College of
  Medicine
Chief, Pediatric Urology
Children's Hospital
Columbus, Ohio

Stanley Kogan, M.D.
Professor of Urology
New York Medical College;
Co-Director
Section of Pediatric Urology
Westchester County Medical Center
New York, New York

Harry Koo, M.D.
Assistant Professor
Section of Urology
University of Michigan
  School of Medicine
Ann Arbor, Michigan

James M. Kozlowski, M.D.
Associate Professor of Urology,
  Surgery, and Tumor Cell Biology
Director, Genitourinary
  Oncology Program
Northwestern University Medical School
Chicago, Illinois

John N. Krieger, M.D.
Professor
Department of Urology
University of Washington
  School of Medicine
Seattle, Washington

Robert M. Levin, M.D.
Research Professor
Division of Urology
Department of Pharmacology
University of Pennsylvania
  School of Medicine
Philadelphia, Pennsylvania

W. Marston Linehan, M.D.
Head, Urologic Oncology Section
Surgery Branch, National Cancer Institute
Bethesda, Maryland

Marguerite C. Lippert, M.D.
Associate Professor
Department of Urology
University of Virginia
  Health Sciences Center
Charlottesville, Virginia

Larry I. Lipshultz, M.D.
Professor
Scott Department of Urology
Baylor College of Medicine
Houston, Texas

Jack W. McAninch, M.D.
Professor and Chief
Department of Urology
University of California
  School of Medicine
San Francisco, California

David L. McCullough, M.D.
Professor and Chairman
Department of Urology
Bowman Gray School of Medicine
Winston-Salem, North Carolina

W. Scott McDougal, M.D.
Professor of Surgery
Department of Urology
Harvard Medical School
Chief of Urology
Massachusetts General Hospital
Boston, Massachusetts

Elspeth M. McDougall, M.D.
Assistant Professor
Division of Urologic Surgery
Washington University
  School of Medicine
St. Louis, Missouri

Edward J. McGuire, M.D.
Professor and Director
Department of Urology
University of Texas Medical School
Houston, Texas

Kevin T. McVary, M.D.
Assistant Professor
Department of Urology
Northwestern University Medical School
Chicago, Illinois

Randall B. Meacham, M.D.
Assistant Professor
Division of Urology
University of Colorado
  Health Sciences Center
Denver, Colorado

Douglas F. Milam, M.D.
Assistant Professor
Department of Urology
Vanderbilt University
  School of Medicine
Nashville, Tennessee

H. Norman Noe, M.D.
Professor
Department of Urology
University of Tennessee
  College of Medicine
Chief of Pediatric Urology
LeBonheur Children's Medical Center
Memphis, Tennessee

Andrew C. Novick, M.D.
Chairman
Department of Urology
Cleveland Clinic Foundation
Cleveland, Ohio

Helen O'Connell, M.D.
Division of Urology
University of Texas Medical School
Houston, Texas

Robert A. Older, M.D.
Associate Professor of Radiology
Chief, Section of Uroradiology
Department of Radiology
University of Virginia
  Health Sciences Center
Charlottesville, Virginia

Jayashree Parekh, M.D.
Assistant Professor
Department of Radiology
University of Virginia
  Health Sciences Center
Charlottesville, Virginia

Raymond E. Poore, M.D.
Department of Urology
Bowman Gray School of Medicine
Winston-Salem, North Carolina

Ronald Rabinowitz, M.D.
Professor of Urology and Pediatrics
University of Rochester School of
  Medicine and Dentistry;
Chief of Pediatric Urology
Strong Memorial Hospital
Chief of Urology
Rochester General Hospital
Rochester, New York

John F. Redman, M.D.
Professor and Chairman
Department of Urology
University of Arkansas for
  Medical Sciences
Chief, Urology Service
University Hospital and
  Arkansas Children's Hospital
Little Rock, Arkansas

Martin I. Resnick, M.D.
Lester Persky Professor and Chairman
Department of Urology
Case Western Reserve University
  School of Medicine
Director, Department of Urology
University Hospitals of Cleveland
Cleveland, Ohio

Michael L. Ritchey, M.D.
Associate Professor of Surgery
  and Pediatrics
Department of Surgery (Urology)
University of Texas Medical School
Chief, Pediatric Urology
Hermann Children's Hospital
Houston, Texas

George T. Rodeheaver, Ph.D.
Research Professor of Plastic Surgery
University of Virginia Health
  Sciences Center
Charlottesville, Virginia

Randall G. Rowland, M.D., Ph.D.
Professor
Department of Urology
Indiana University School of Medicine
Indianapolis, Indiana

Grannum R. Sant, M.D.
Professor and Vice-Chairman
Department of Urology
Tufts University School of Medicine
Boston, Massachusetts

Anthony J. Schaeffer, M.D.
Herman L. Kretschmer Professor
  and Chairman
Department of Urology
Northwestern University Medical School
Chicago, Illinois

Curtis A. Sheldon, M.D.
Associate Professor of Surgery
Division of Urology
University of Cincinnati
  College of Medicine;
Director, Pediatric Urology
Children's Hospital Medical Center
Cincinnati, Ohio

Grahame H. H. Smith, M.D.
Formerly, Fellow
Department of Pediatric Surgery
The Children's Hospital of Philadelphia
Philadelphia, Pennsylvania;
Royal Alexandra Children's Hospital
Sydney, Australia

Joseph A. Smith, Jr., M.D.
William L. Bray Professor and Chairman
Department of Urology
Vanderbilt University
  School of Medicine
Nashville, Tennessee

Brent W. Snow, M.D.
Associate Professor of Urology/Pediatrics
University of Utah
  Health Sciences Center
Salt Lake City, Utah

Howard M. Snyder III, M.D.
Division of Urology
Children's Hospital of of Philadelphia
Philadelphia, Pennsylvania

R. Ernest Sosa, M.D.
Associate Professor
Department of Urology
Cornell University Medical College
New York, New York

J. Patrick Spirnack, M.D.
Associate Professor
Department of Urology
Case Western Reserve University
  School of Medicine;
Director of Urology
Metrohealth Medical Center
Cleveland, Ohio

William D. Steers, M.D.
Chairman and
J.Y. Gillenwater Professor of Urology
Department of Urology
University of Virginia
  Health Sciences Center
Charlottesville, Virginia

Gerald Sufrin, M.D.
Professor and Chairman
Department of Urology
State University of New York
  at Buffalo
School of Medicine and
  Biomedical Sciences
Buffalo, New York

Charles D. Teates, M.D.
Professor
Department of Radiology
University of Virginia
  Health Sciences Center
Charlottesville, Virginia

Charles J. Tegtmeyer, M.D.
Professor of Radiology and Anatomy
Director, Division of Angiography,
  Interventional Radiology, and
  Special Procedures
Department of Radiology
University of Virginia
  Health Sciences Center
Charlottesville, Virginia

John G. Thacker, Ph.D.
Professor of Mechanical Engineering
Department of Mechanical and
  Aerospace Engineering
University of Virginia
  Health Sciences Center
Charlottesville, Virginia

Joseph G. Trapasso, M.D.
Department of Urology
Graduate Hospital
Philadelphia, Pennsylvania

E. Darracott Vaughan, Jr., M.D.
James J. Colt Professor of Urology
Department of Urology
Cornell University Medical College
New York, New York

Robert L. Vogelzang, M.D.
Associate Professor
Department of Radiology
Northwestern University Medical School
Chicago, Illinois

R. Dixon Walker III, M.D.
Professor of Surgery
Division of Urology
University of Florida College
  of Medicine;
Chief of Pediatric Urology
Shands Hospital
Gainesville, Florida

Alan J. Wein, M.D.
Professor and Chairman
Division of Urology
University of Pennsylvania
  School of Medicine
Chief of Urology
Hospital of the University
  of Pennsylvania
Philadelphia, Pennsylvania

Jeffrey P. Weiss, M.D.
Clinical Associate Professor of Urology
Temple University School of Medicine
Philadelphia, Pennsylvania

Robert M. Weiss, M.D.
Professor and Chief
Section of Urology
Yale University School of Medicine
New Haven, Connecticut

B. Dale Wilson, M.D.
Assistant Professor
Department of Dermatology
Roswell Park Cancer Institute
State University of New York
  at Buffalo
School of Medicine and
  Biomedical Sciences
Buffalo, New York

Julia A. Woods, B.A.
Department of Plastic Surgery
University of Virginia
  Health Sciences Center
Charlottesville, Virginia

Arthur W. Wyker, Jr., M.D.
Urology Associates
Kingsport, Tennessee

Stephen A. Zderic, M.D.
Assistant Professor
Division of Urology
University of Pennsylvania
  School of Medicine
Attending Surgeon
The Children's Hospital of Philadelphia
Philadelphia, Pennsylvania

CONTENTS

1
Anatomy of the Genitourinary System
John F. Redman

1. As a surgeon frees a large retroperitoneal mass from the dorsal aspect of the right side of the upper abdomen, the dissecting hand will encounter the junctures of the diaphragm with the posterior abdominal wall muscles. These junctures are termed:

    a. the triangular and coronary ligaments.
    b. costovertebral ligaments.
    c. medial and lateral lumbocostal arcs.
    d. crura of the diaphragm.
    e. Cooper's ligaments.

    Correct Answer: c   Reference Page: 5
    Rationale: The diaphragm in the dorsum of the retroperitoneum crosses over the psoas major and quadratus lumborum muscles as fibrous arcs termed respectively the medial and lateral lumbocostal arcs or arcuate ligaments. The arcs are the lumbar origins of the diaphragm.

2. The retroperitoneal connective tissue which forms Gerota's fascia and contains the ureter and spermatic vessels and encases the pelvic organs is termed:

    a. Denonvilliers' fascia.
    b. inner stratum of retroperitoneal connective tissue.
    c. transversalis fascia.
    d. intermediate stratum of retroperitoneal connective tissue.
    e. outer stratum of retroperitoneal connective tissue.

    Correct Answer: d   Reference Page: 10
    Rationale: The intermediate stratum of retroperitoneal connective tissue is the fat-laden connective tissue which lies between the outer stratum (transversalis fascia) and the inner stratum (the supporting connective tissues of the retroperitoneum). Its condensations form Gerota's fascia and the supports and ligaments of the pelvic organs.

3. As the urologist develops the incision for a radical perineal prostatectomy, the dissection on either side of the midline opens the wedge-shaped space termed the ischiorectal fossa, which is located between what muscles?

    a. Obturator internus and levator ani

b.   Rectourethralis and transverse perineal
c.   Ischiocavernosus and levator ani
d.   Coccygeus and transverse perineal
e.   Piriformis and transverse perineal

Correct Answer: a   Reference Page: 18
Rationale: The fat-filled space termed the ischiorectal fossa is wedge-shaped owing to its position between the relatively flat obturator internus muscle and the funnel shaped levator ani muscle. Development of this space allows for isolation and the subsequent division of the central tendon of the perineum which exposes Denonvilliers' fascia.

4.   **In the course of a nephrolithotomy, the urologist cuts across the region of the juncture of the renal cortex and the pyramid near the papilla and encounters brisk bleeding. What vessel has been cut?**

a.   Segmental artery
b.   Arcuate artery
c.   Interlobar artery
d.   Interlobular artery
e.   Vasa Recta

Correct Answer: c   Reference Page: 26
Rationale: The segmental renal artery branches into 2 or 3 interlobar arteries which enter the cortex on either side of the pyramids. Injury to the interlobar artery will render the parenchyma thus supplied ischemic since all renal arteries are end arteries.

5.   **A patient has an invasive transitional cell bladder lesion located in the anterior superior aspect of the bladder. Lymph nodes to be first suspected of involvement would be located in which group?**

a.   Hypogastric group
b.   External iliac group
c.   Internal iliac group
d.   Pudendal group
e.   Lateral sacral group

Correct Answer: b   Reference Page: 36
Rationale: Lymphatics follow the vasculature of an organ. The anterior superior aspect of the bladder was developmentally supplied by branches of the umbilical artery, which becomes obliterated to become the medial umbilical ligament. The persistent lymphatics follow the ligament and course along the remnant of the umbilical artery to terminate in nodes of the middle chain of the external iliac group.

6.   A 25-year-old man has undergone a right radical orchiectomy for a testicular mass which on pathological examination is determined to be a nonseminomatous testis cancer. Considering the lymphatic drainage of the right testis, the most common site of tumor deposition would be the:

a.   right paracaval zone.
b.   right precaval zone.
c.   right iliac zone.
d.   right suprahilar zone.
e.   interaortocaval zone.

Correct Answer: e   Reference Page: 44

Rationale: The work of Donohue and associates on the distribution of nodal metastases in nonseminomatous testis tumors clearly established the lymphatic drainage of the testes. The interaortocaval zone just below the left renal vein is the most common site (93%) of tumor deposition of right-sided testis tumors.

7.   A patient is found to have a large adrenal mass extending behind the right lobe of the liver. The surgeon wishes to free the liver from the abdominal side wall for better visualization of the mass. To effect such exposure, the surgeon should incise the:

a.   right triangular ligament.
b.   falciform ligament.
c.   hepatogastric ligament.
d.   ligamentum teres.
e.   hepatic flexure.

Correct Answer: a   Reference Page: 58

Rationale: To reflect the liver from the right side of the abdominal wall, the surgeon must first incise the right triangular ligament which represents the peritoneal reflection from the abdominal side wall onto the liver. This is followed by incision medially of the contiguous upper and lower coronary ligaments.

2
Standard Diagnostic Considerations
Wade Bushman and Arthur W. Wyker, Jr.

1.   A 72-year-old white male with a history of congestive heart failure, peripheral edema, and an enlarged prostate complains of nocturia q 1-2 hours. He denies frequency, hesitancy, diminished force of stream or sensation of incomplete emptying. The first step in his evaluation should be:

   a. cystometrogram.
   b. trial of anticholinergic medication.
   c. voiding diary.
   d. cystoscopy.
   e. flow rate.

   Correct Answer: c   Reference Page: 63
   Rationale: This patient presents with isolated nocturia without daytime frequency or obstructive symptoms. Situational frequency such as this may be explained by increased urine production. In this case, the patient's symptoms may be due to nocturnal mobilization of edema fluid. This is most clearly demonstrated by a 24-hour voiding diary.

2.   Which of the following statements about urge incontinence is false?

   a. It can be classified as a failure to store urine.
   b. It is commonly seen in stroke patients.
   c. It can only be reliably diagnosed with a cystometrogram.
   d. The most common cause is idiopathic detrusor instability.
   e. A detailed history and a 24-hour voiding diary are usually sufficient to make the diagnosis.

   Correct Answer: c   Reference Page: 65
   Rationale: In patients with urge incontinence the history of episodic urinary leakage in association with a precipitous urge is usually characteristic. While a cystometrogram may demonstrate uninhibited detrusor activity during bladder filling this study has a significant incidence of false negative and false positive results and it is not necessary for the diagnosis.

3.   **A 68-year-old man presents with microscopic hematuria. The most likely etiology of hematuria in the patient is:**

   a.   kidney stones.
   b.   BPH.
   c.   UTI.
   d.   bladder tumor.
   e.   glomerulonephritis.

   Correct Answer: b   Reference Page: 67
   Rationale: BPH is the most common cause of microscopic hematuria in this age group.

4.   **Which of the following statements about upper urinary tract pain is true?**

   a.   It is directly proportional to the degree of distension evident on IVP.
   b.   It occurs predominantly in a mid-abdominal distribution.
   c.   Distension of the upper ureter may cause referred pain to the contralateral testis.
   d.   A normal IVP during a pain episode rules out GU tract obstruction as the cause of pain.
   e.   Distension of the renal capsule causes intermittent colicky pain.

   Correct Answer: d   Reference Page: 67
   Rationale: Pain with obstruction is caused by increased intraluminal pressure. Since increased pressure produces distension, the absence of distension on IVP effectively rules out obstruction as the cause of urinary tract pain. Long-term obstruction may produce marked distension without significant pain. Distension of the renal capsule more typically causes steady non-colicky pain.

5.   **Which of the following patients is least likely to exhibit renal insufficiency?**

   a.   A 58-year-old female with locally advanced ovarian cancer and bilateral hydronephrosis
   b.   A 70-year-old diabetic man with a post void residual urine volume of 1500 cc
   c.   A 72-year-old man with urinary retention and bilateral hydronephrosis
   d.   A 38-year-old man with right renal agenesis and an obstructing 4 mm stone at hydronephrosis
   e.   A 50-year-old female with a 10 mm left UPJ stone and severe left hydrone-phrosis

Correct Answer: e   Reference Page: 69
Rationale: The patient described in E is the only patient with a unilateral process. The compensatory function of the presumably normal contralateral kidney would be expected to maintain normal renal function.

6.   **A 58-year-old recently divorced man presents with a 2-month history of impotence. Which of the following signs and symptoms points to a psychogenic etiology?**

    a.   Normal serum testosterone
    b.   Normal libido
    c.   Episodic difficulty achieving erection with a new partner
    d.   Normal peripheral pulses
    e.   No history of hypertension or diabetes mellitus

Correct Answer: c   Reference Page: 69
Rationale: An episodic pattern of difficulty achieving an erection is more typical of a psychogenic rather than organic etiology.

7.   **A 38-year-old white female presents with several day history of frequency, nocturia and dysuria. Her urine contains only occasional WBCs. Culture of urine obtained by catheterization reveals 10^4 cfu/ml _E. coli_ and a 3-day course of antibiotics relieves her symptoms. This case shows:**

    a.   the patient's irritative symptoms may be unrelated to the presence of infection.
    b.   the absence of pyuria effectively rules out infection.
    c.   catheterization can introduce significant bacteriuria.
    d.   a urine culture is necessary to rule out the presence of infection.
    e.   greater than 10^5 cfu/ml is the threshold for a significant symptomatic urinary tract infection.

Correct Answer: c   Reference Page: 76
Rationale: Urinary tract infections may occur in the absence of significant pyuria and may only be effectively ruled out with a urine culture. While a positive culture is generally considered to be greater than 10^5 cfu/ml on a voided specimen as few as 10^3 cfu/ml may present significant bacteriuria in a catheterized specimen.

3A
Excretory Urography

Robert A. Older, Charles D. Kellum,
Loulie M. Fisher, Chalres J. Tegtmeyer

1. **The major advantage of using nonionic iodinating contrast media as opposed to ionic iodinated contrast media is:**

   a. decreased incidence of nephrotoxicity.
   b. decreased cost.
   c. improvement in the quality of the urogram.
   d. significant reduction in moderate and severe contrast reactions.
   e. more widespread availability.

   Correct Answer: d   Reference Pages: 86-87
   Rationale: Nonionic contrast media not only have significantly reduced physiologic responses such as warmth, flushing and nausea, but also have a well documented decrease in all forms of allergic reactions. The decrease in these adverse effects as well as the physiologic effects is thought to be primarily due to the reduced osmolality of the nonionic agents as compared to the ionic contrast.

2. **The indicated therapy for a contrast reaction consisting of severe bronchospasm and/or laryngeal edema with hypotension is:**

   a. immediate treatment with corticosteroids.
   b. immediate treatment with antihistamines.
   c. immediate treatment with intravenous epinephrine with a slow push of 1 ml of 1:10,000 dilution.
   d. immediate treatment with subcutaneous epinephrine in a dose of 0.1 to 0.2 ml of 1:1000.
   e. atropine.

   Correct Answer: c   Reference Page: 85
   Rationale: Once a severe reaction to iodinated contrast has occurred, steroids are of little benefit in immediate treatment. Benadryl may prevent further release of histamine, but does not counteract the reaction which is already occurring. Epinephrine is the treatment of choice for a severe reaction such as described above. Because a severe reaction may rapidly progress to vascular collapse, it is important to administer the epinephrine intravenously to be certain that it reaches the central circulation. Absorption of subcutaneous epinephrine can be inconsistent in this

setting. The epinephrine is given as a 1 to 10,000 dilution and should be given slowly. One ml is sufficient for the initial dose.

3.   **The optimal time for visualizing the renal parenchyma during urography is at:**

   a.   5 minutes postinjection.
   b.   10 minutes postinjection.
   c.   8 minutes postinjection.
   d.   immediately following completion of contrast injection.
   e.   30 minutes postinjection.

Correct Answer: d   Reference Page: 89
Rationale: The nephrogram depends on the concentration of iodinated contrast material in the circulating blood and this is maximal immediately following the bolus injection of contrast media. Afterwards there is normally a progressive decline in the nephrogram.

4.   **Technical factors play a major role in determining whether or not a urogram is of high quality. Which of the following technical aspects is of most value in detecting a parenchymal lesion such as renal cell carcinoma?**

   a.   Oblique views
   b.   Post-void films
   c.   Upright views
   d.   Tomography
   e.   Abdominal compression

Correct Answer: d   Reference Page: 94
Rationale: Tomography is one of the most important technical factors in performing urography and should be available in essentially all studies. Tomography allows us to select a focal zone for visualization and blurs out surrounding structures such as bowel content. This vastly improves the visualization of the renal parenchyma and therefore the detection of parenchymal abnormalities such as masses.

3B
Renal Arteriography and Computed Tomography
Stuart S. Howards and Robert L. Vogelzang

1. **The nephrogram of a renal arteriogram consists of the following phases:**

    a. cortical arteriogram, glomerulogram, cortical nephrogram, and general nephrogram.
    b. cortical arteriogram and cortical nephrogram.
    c. nephrogram.
    d. cortical arteriogram, cortical nephrogram, and general nephrogram.
    e. cortical arteriogram and general nephrogram.

    Correct Answer: a   Reference Page: 101

    Rationale: The phases correspond to the sequence in which the contrast enters each functional unit of the kidney. It is clinically important to look for a nephrogram early after the injection of contrast.

2. **To achieve a high degree of accuracy in identifying a renal cyst with a CT scan, the following criteria should be met:**

    a. Uniform water density contents with attenuation no greater than 30 HU; rounded or oval mass without a perceptible wall; absence of contrast enhancement.
    b. Uniform water density contents with attenuation no greater than 30 HU; peripheral location; absence of contrast enhancement.
    c. Uniform water density contents with attenuation no greater than 20 HU; rounded or oval mass without a perceptible wall; absence of contrast enhancement.
    d. Uniform water density contents with attenuation no greater than 30 HU; peripheral location; absence of contrast enhancement.
    e. Uniform water density contents with attenuation no greater than 30 HU; rounded or oval mass without a perceptible wall; absence of contrast enhancement; peripheral location.

    Correct Answer: c   Reference Page: 118

    Rationale: These criteria make the identification of renal cysts rather straightforward in most cases. It is important to look at the images in an organized, systematic fashion to avoid mistakes.

3. **The characteristics of xanthigranulomatous pyelonephritis on renal arteriogram are:**

a. decreased central vascularity, crisp definition, hydronephrosis, and well-defined corticomedullary junction.
b. decreased central vascularity, crisp definition, hydronephrosis, and poorly defined corticomedullary junction.
c. decreased central vascularity, ill-defined mass, hydronephrosis, and well-defined corticomedullary junction.
d. decreased central vascularity, ill-defined mass, hydronephrosis, and poorly defined corticomedullary junction; homogeneous nephrogram.
e. decreased central vascularity, ill-defined mass, hydronephrosis, and poorly defined corticomedullary junction.

Correct Answer: e   Reference Page: 108

Rationale: Xanthogranulomatous pyelonephritis is an uncommon disease. Nevertheless, it is important to make the diagnosis preoperatively if possible. These criteria are useful but not foolproof.

3C
Magnetic Resonance Imaging
Peter Choyke

1. **Which one of the following statements regarding the appearance of urinary tract structures on MR is *false*?**

    a.   On T1 weighted images fat is bright; urine is dark.

    b.   On T2 weighted images fat is bright; urine is bright.

    c.   On fat suppressed T2 weighted images fat is dark; urine is bright.

    d.   All MR pulse sequences take at least one minute to perform and thus are susceptible to motion artifact.

    e.   Surface coils are advantageous because they increase signal and decrease noise.

Correct Answer: d   Reference Pages: 147, 148

Rationale: New fast gradient echo and echo-planar pulse sequences can be obtained within several seconds easily within the ability of a patient to hold his breath. On T1 and T2 weighted images fat is generally bright unless fat suppression is employed. Urine (and most renal cysts and renal tumors) are dark on T1 weighted scans and bright on T2 weighted scans regardless of the addition of fat suppression. Surface coils increase the "signal to noise" ratio in MR by both increasing signal (the coil is closer to the target) and decreasing noise (extraneous signals absorbed by the body are not received by the coil).

2. **Regarding the use of gadolinium-chelates in MRI:**

    a.   Iodinated contrast media and gadolinium chelates have similar rates of allergic reactions.

    b.   Iodinated contrast media and gadolinium chelates have a similar rate of nephrotoxicity.

    c.   Gadolinium-enhanced MRI can be used in place of contrast enhanced CT for renal masses.

    d.   As gadolinium concentrates in the urinary system it gives a brighter signal.

    e.   Gadolinium is contraindicated for patents on dialysis.

Correct Answer: c   Reference Pages: 147, 150

Rationale: Gadolinium chelates differ from iodinated contrast media because they have a lower frequency of allergic reactions and nephrotoxicity. Gadolinium chelates can be given to patients on dialysis but the patient should undergo dialysis soon after the MRI. As gadolinium concentrates in the urinary tract, particularly in the bladder, it first increases and then decreases in signal intensity. This is best seen in the bladder (the "oreo cookie" sign) where the layers contrast: unopacified urine on top (black), intermediate concentration of gadolinium chelate in the middle (white) and high concentration of gadolinium in the dependent portion of the bladder (black).

Gadolinium-enhanced MRI can be used in place of contrast enhanced CT for renal masses in patients with allergies to iodinated contrast media or renal dysfunction.

3. **Indications for MRI in the genitourinary tract include all *except*:**

   a. evaluating the inferior vena cava for tumor thrombus when staging renal carcinoma.
   b. differentiating adrenal adenomas and nonadenomas.
   c. differentiating oncocytomas from renal carcinoma and angiomyolipomas.
   d. identifying pheochromocytomas and paragangliomas.
   e. evaluating the renal artery for stenosis in patients with poor renal function.

Correct Answer: c   Reference Pages: 152, 153, 155
Rationale: The major indications for MRI in the kidney are: staging renal cancers for venous invasion, differentiating cystic and solid renal masses and evaluating the renal artery with MR angiography in patients with renal dysfunction. However, MR cannot differentiate oncocytomas from renal cancers. While fat components of angiomyolipomas can be identified on MRI, CT is preferred for this task.

The major indications for MRI in the adrenal are in identifying pheochromocytomas which are *usually* intensely bright on T2 weighted images, and differentiating adenomas from nonadenomas on the basis of fat content on chemical shift MRI.

4. **The MRI of the urinary tract:**

   a. can be substituted for the intravenous pyelogram to evaluate the urothelial tract.
   b. can more accurately stage bladder cancers than cystoscopic biopsy.
   c. is no more accurate than CT for detecting lymphadenopathy.
   d. is limited to the same degree as CT by the presence of stainless steel surgical clips in the retroperitoneum.
   e. includes enlargement and abnormal signal intensity as criteria for abnormal lymph nodes.

Correct Answer: c   Reference Pages: 158-159
Rationale: MRI relies on the same criterion as CT, enlargement, to detect abnormal lymph nodes. Answer e is incorrect because signal intensity of lymph nodes has proven to be unreliable. MRI does not have the same spatial resolution as IVP for detecting urothelial malignancies. The accuracy of MRI for staging bladder cancers is under study; currently one cannot state that MR can more accurately stage bladder cancers. MRI is less influenced by the presence of stainless steel clips, which are nonmagnetic, than is CT. Ferromagnetic material (e.g., shrapnel), however, causes more severe defects on MRI than on CT.

5. **Which statement regarding MRI of the prostate and testicle is *not* true?**

    a. Endorectal coil MRI of the prostate is superior to body coil MRI because of the higher resolution.

    b. Invasion of the seminal vesicles appears as a low signal intensity defect within the normally high signal intensity seminal vesicles.

    c. Better image quality may result from combining endorectal coils and surface phased array coils.

    d. Endorectal coil MRI reliably predicts microscopic extension of prostate cancer outside the capsule.

    e. The normal testicles are high in signal intensity on T2 weighted MRI.

Correct Answer: d   Reference Pages: 150-151

Rationale: All of the choices are correct except d. While endorectal coil MRI is generally reliable for macroscopic transcapsular extension of prostate cancer, it does not have sufficient resolution to identify microscopic extension.

3D
Ultrasound

J. Patrick Spirnak and Martin I. Resnick

1. **All of the following statements about ultrasound are true *except*:**

   a. The frequency of sound waves used for medical purposes is between 2 and 10 million cycles per second.
   b. Frequency is the number of times the ultrasound wave is repeated per second.
   c. As the frequency of the transducer is increased, depth of penetration increases.
   d. Resolution is dependent on transducer frequency.
   e. The greater the difference in acoustic impedance between two media, the greater the amount of sound reflected back from the interface.

   Correct Answer: c   Reference Pages: 166-167

   Rationale: As the frequency of the transducer increases, resolution increases but depth of penetration decreases. Picking the appropriate transducer is critical for a successful ultrasonic exam. Scrotal and transrectal ultrasounds typically use transducers of 7.5 MHz, while kidney exams are usually performed with 3.5 MHz transducers.

2. **All of the following may cause a false positive diagnosis of hydronephrosis *except*:**

   a. extrarenal pelvis.
   b. high urinary output.
   c. child with a full bladder.
   d. a hemorrhagic cyst.
   e. a parapelvic cyst.

   Correct Answer: d   Reference Page: 173

   Rationale: Ultrasound approaches a sensitivity of nearly 100% for the diagnosis of hydronephrosis. Other lesions that can be mistaken for hydronephrosis include calyceal diverticulum, congenital megacalycosis, and parenchymal renal cysts. In children, the collecting system is easily distensible and therefore, a repeat study may need to be performed after the child voids. False negative results can occur with dehydration, acute obstruction, forniceal rupture which decompresses the collecting system or peripelvic inflammation or tumor which prevents dilation of the collecting system. A hemorrhagic cyst should not be confused with hydronephrosis as it will have variable echogenicity whereas urine is anechoic.

3.   **A nonopaque renal pelvis filling defect is seen on IVP. Ultrasound reveals dense echoes and acoustic shadowing. The most likely diagnosis is:**

a.   blood clot.
b.   tumor.
c.   sloughed renal papilla.
d.   uric acid stone.
e.   crossing vessel.

Correct Answer: d   Reference Page: 173
Rationale: Ultrasound can be very helpful in differentiating nonopaque or poorly calcified renal calculi from soft tissue filling defects in the renal pelvis. The renal calculus completely reflects sound waves, casting a characteristic "echo free" acoustic shadow behind the stone. Other nonopaque stones are mucoid matrix and xanthine calculi.

4.   **Clinical applications of prostate ultrasonography include all of the following *except*:**

a.   prostatic volume determination.
b.   aid in prostate biopsy.
c.   placement of interstitial radiation seeds.
d.   screening for prostate cancer.
e.   evaluation of the prostate after abdominal perineal resection.

Correct Answer: d   Reference Pages: 183-186
Rationale: The ultrasonic characteristics of carcinoma of the prostate are variable and not very specific. Lesions can be hypoechoic, hyperechoic, isoechoic or mixed echogenicity. Benign processes, such as infarct or small nodules of benign prostatic hyperplasia, can have similar characteristics. Therefore, ultrasound is not very sensitive nor specific in detecting prostate cancer lesions and it should not be used to determine which patient should undergo biopsy.

5.   **Which statement about renal ultrasound is *true*?**

a.   Ultrasonic characteristics of a renal cyst include spherical shape, thin walls, anechoic, and anterior wall enhancement.
b.   The ultrasonic diagnosis of a cystic lesion is more accurate than a solid lesion.
c.   Hypoechogenicity is the most distinguishing feature of angiomyolipoma.
d.   The majority of fetal kidneys can be detected by 12 weeks gestation.
e.   Patients with end stage renal failure have small, hypoechoic kidneys.

Correct Answer: b   Reference Pages: 171-172

Rationale: Ultrasound approaches 100% sensitive for the diagnosis of renal cysts. It can detect cysts as small as 1 to 2 mm. In contrast, solid lesions typically are not accurately diagnosed until 1 to 2 cm in size. As a result, there is an approximately 14% false negative rate for ultrasonic detection of solid masses.

6.   **An 18-year-old boy presents with a painful, tender scrotum. Which diagnosis will ultrasound be most helpful in excluding:**

    a.   malignancy.
    b.   epididimorchitis.
    c.   testicular torsion.
    d.   traumatic testicular disruption.
    e.   rhabdomyosarcoma of the spermatic cord

Correct Answer: e   Reference Pages: 178-179

Rationale: Scrotal ultrasound is most helpful in distinguishing intratesticular from paratesticular lesions. All of the testicular lesions above may appear inhomogeneous, hypoechoic.

7.   **The ultrasonic appearance of prostate cancer is:**

    a.   isoechoic.
    b.   hyperechoic.
    c.   hypoechoic.
    d.   mixed echogenicity.
    e.   all of the above.

Correct Answer: e   Reference Page: 178

Rationale: The ultrasonic appearance of prostate cancer is highly variable, and therefore ultrasound is not very specific in the detection of prostate cancer.

3E
Nuclide Studies

Barbara Y. Croft, Judith M. Joyce,
Jayashree Parekh, Charles D. Teates

1. **What kind of examination potentially confers the highest radiation dose?**

   a. A nuclear medicine examination

   b. X-ray fluoroscopy

   c. Intravenous pyelogram

Correct Answer: b   Reference Page: 196

Rationale: Fluoroscopy doses are the highest; the dose may be 10 rad/min for a minute of exposure. The mean exposure from an IVP is 3 R, which includes about 0.6 rads to the female gonads. The nuclear medicine examination may give up to 4.2 rads to the bladder wall of an adult for the Tc-99m glucoheptonate examination or 1.7 rads to the bladder for the more usual Tc-99m DTPA examination and no more than 0.2 rads to the gonads for any of the nuclear medicine examinations.

2. **What radionuclide is recommended for use in the severely oliguric or anuric patients?**

   a. Tc-99m MAG_3

   b. I-131 hippuran

   c. Tc-99m DTPA

   d. Tc-99m Glucoheptonate

   e. Tc-99m DMSA

Correct Answer: a   Reference Page: 205

Rationale: Tc-99m MAG_3 or I-131 hippuran is recommended because Tc-99m DTPA or Tc-99m GH poorly visualize the system. X-ray contrast is not indicated both because of potentially adverse effects on the patient who cannot excrete the material and because the kidneys will not be visualized. The Tc-99m MAG_3 is preferred over I-131 hippuran because of the better count rate.

3. **Different curves of activity vs. time are expected in the case of renal imaging with Tc-99m DTPA and subsequent furosemide imaging. Describe the shape of the curve for the obstructed patient.**

   a. Slowly falling, with sharper fall post-furosemide

   b. Rising, then falling sharply post-furosemide

   c. Rising, then continuing to rise post-furosemide

   d. Rising and plateauing post-furosemide

Correct Answer: c   Reference Page: 207

Rationale: Four patterns are possible. A slowly falling curve, with sharper decline after furosemide, indicates a normal kidney with no obstruction. A rising curve, which turns around and falls after furosemide, indicates no obstruction also; the increased volume running through the system dilutes the urine and pushes it out. A rising curve which continues to rise post-furosemide indicates obstruction; added volume does not cause the system to drain. A rising and plateauing pattern, seemingly unaffected by furosemide, is indeterminate, indicating poor renal function and poor response to furosemide and/or a large, atonic hydronephrotic sac.

4. **Describe the radioactive agent and the response in captopril renography.**

   a. Tc-99m DTPA; increase in function after captopril indicates drug-controllable hypertension
   b. Tc-99m MAG$_3$; increase in function after captopril indicates compensated tubular secretion
   c. I-131 hippuran; decrease in function after captopril indicates intrarenal compensation
   d. Tc-99m DTPA; decrease in function after captopril indicates renal artery stenosis

Correct Answer: d   Reference Page: 212

Rationale: Tc-99m DTPA would seem to be the best agent because it is excreted by glomerular filtration, the process most affected; Tc-99m MAG$_3$ seems to give good results, however. If the renogram is performed with and without captopril administration, one can observe if there is a change. A change in renal function for the worse in one kidney indicates renal artery stenosis as a cause for renal hypertension.

4
Biology of Wound Repair and Infection

Richard A. Edlich, Julia A. Woods,
George T. Rodeheaver, John G. Thacker

1. **The optimal time for delayed primary closure of contaminated wounds is on or after:**

a. 12 hours after wounding.
b. 24 hours after wounding.
c. 48 hours after wounding.
d. 72 hours after wounding.
e. 96 hours after wounding.

Correct Answer: e   Reference Page: 228

Rationale: When a wound is left open, there is a dramatic increase in vascular permeability that results in the development of a thick inflammatory exudate on the wound surface. This fibrinous coagulum serves as a plug in the transected ends of lymphatics in the wound, thereby becoming an obstacle to the invasion of bacteria and enhancing the resistance of an open wound to systemic sepsis. On or after the fourth postoperative day the margins of the open wound without devitalized tissue can be approximated with minimum risk of infection.

2. **The minimum infective dose of aerobic bacteria in adipose tissue is:**

a. 10^3 per gram of tissue.
b. 10^4 per gram of tissue.
c. 10^5 per gram of tissue.
d. 10^6 per gram of tissue.
e. 10^7 per gram of tissue.

Correct Answer: d   Reference Page: 237

Rationale: A critical number of bacteria appear to be necessary to elicit infection in soft tissue wounds. In experimental animals the infective dose of obligate and facultative aerobic bacteria in wounds is 10^6 bacteria or greater per gram of tissue. When the aerobic bacterial counts are below this level, the wounds will heal consistently without infection.

3. **A dressing that prevents exogenous bacterial contamination should cover a wound approximated by percutaneous sutures for at least:**

a.   12 hours.
b.   24 hours.
c.   48 hours.
d.   72 hours.
e.   96 hours.

Correct Answer: c   Reference Page: 229
Rationale: Experimental studies have demonstrated that as they heal, sutured wounds were susceptible to infection after surface contamination during the first 48 hours after wound closure. Surface contamination on the third postoperative day did not produce gross infection in the sutured wound. This susceptibility to infection during the early postoperative period confirms the apparent value of dressings until 48 hours postoperatively to protect the sutured wound from surface contamination.

4. **Dead space closure between the cut edges of subcutaneous (adipose) tissue should be accomplished by:**

a.   interrupted absorbable synthetic sutures.
b.   interrupted absorbable gut sutures.
c.   interrupted nonabsorbable braided sutures.
d.   interrupted nonabsorbable monofilament sutures.
e.   no suture.

Correct Answer: e   Reference Page: 271
Rationale: Sutural closure of the adipose tissue below the skin should be avoided. Obliteration of this potential dead space between the cut edge of adipose tissue by even the least reactive suture increases the incidence of infection.

5. **Closure of peritoneum is best accomplished with:**

a.   a continuous synthetic monofilament absorbable suture.
b.   an interrupted synthetic monofilament absorbable suture.
c.   a continuous synthetic monofilament nonabsorbable suture.
d.   an interrupted synthetic monofilament nonabsorbable suture.
e.   no suture.

Correct Answer: e   Reference Page: 235
Rationale: Peritoneal repair can be complicated by the development of intraabdominal adhesions, which are the most common cause of acute intestinal obstruction. In peritoneal repair, careful avoidance of all foreign materials is mandatory. No attempt should be made to reconstruct a peritoneal defect; the peritoneal portion of abdominal incisions should never be approximated by sutures.

6. **Hair removal around the perineum and genitalia is best accomplished by a(n):**

a.   razor 24 hours before surgery.
b.   razor immediately before surgery.
c.   depilatory 24 hours before surgery.
d.   electric clipper 24 hours before surgery.
e.   electric clipper immediately before surgery.

Correct Answer: e   Reference Page: 246

Rationale: Research has demonstrated that the technique and timing of hair removal has a considerable influence on the incidence of postoperative infection. Clipping the hair the morning of the operation is associated with significantly fewer infections than were encountered in patients whose hair was removed either by electric clippers the night before the operation or by shaving. A depilatory should not be used near a patient's eyes or genitalia because it can cause serious irritation to these tissues.

7.   **Percutaneous sutures should be removed before the __________ postoperative day to prevent the formation of needle puncture scars.**

a.   second
b.   fourth
c.   eighth
d.   twelfth
e.   sixteenth

Correct Answer: c   Reference Page: 231

Rationale: With the organization of scar epithelium, downward growth of epithelial cells occurs not only at the incision but also at any interruption of the skin, such as suture tracts. These epithelial cells undergo cellular differentiation, inducing an intense inflammatory reaction and scar formation. If the percutaneous sutures are removed before the eighth postoperative day, the invasive spurs of epithelium regress, leaving no discernible deformity.

8.   **The only skin wound cleaner that can be safely poured in the patient's wound as well as eye, without irritation is:**

a.   pleuronic polyol F-68.
b.   chlorhexidine.
c.   iodophore.
d.   tincture of iodine.
e.   aqueous iodine.

Correct Answer: a   Reference Page: 247

Rationale: Pleuronic polyol F-68, a nonionic surfactant, is an excellent substitute for toxic detergents. Unlike all other commercial scrub solutions, the surfactant is so innocuous that it "does not bring tears to a baby's eye."

5
Urinary Tract Infections
Anthony J. Schaeffer

1. **What is the primary virulence factor for uropathogenic E. coli?**

   a. Bacterial adherence
   b. Hemolysin
   c. Antigen
   d. Lipopolysaccharide
   e. Flagella

   Correct Answer: a   Reference Page: 291
   Rationale: It is well established that bacterial adherence to epithelial cells is an essential step in the initiation of urinary tract infections. If the bacteria cannot adhere then subsequent colonization and invasion will not occur. Bacteria adhere to specific binding sites in the urinary tract and their ability to adhere is associated with infection of the urethra, bladder, or kidney.

2. **The drug of choice for uncomplicated acute cystitis is:**

   a. Nitrofurantoin.
   b. TMP/SMX.
   c. Cefallxin.
   d. Noroxin.
   e. Ampicillin.

   Correct Answer: b   Reference Page: 304
   Rationale: TMP-SMX offers the best spectrum of activity at the lowest cost. Noroxin is more effective but too expensive. Bacterial resistance to the other drugs is significantly higher than to TMP/SMX.

3. **What is the primary risk factor for recurrent urinary tract infections in women?**

   a. Vaginal cell receptivity
   b. Diaphragm use
   c. Sexual intercourse
   d. Increasing age
   e. Menopausal status

Correct Answer: a   Reference Page: 295

Rationale: Adherence of bacteria to the vaginal mucosa with subsequent colonization is a critical step in ascending urinary tract infections. Women who are susceptible to infection have increased receptivity for bacteria and during periods of remission have a degree of receptivity for bacteria which approaches that of healthy women who are not colonized with bacteria and do not get urinary tract infections.

4. **When should a woman who is on empiric antimicrobial therapy for acute pyelonephritis undergo radiologic evaluation?**

    a. Immediately
    b. If febrile for longer than 3 days
    c. If there is a history of recurrent urinary tract infections
    d. If blood cultures are positive
    e. After the infection subsides

Correct Answer: b   Reference Page: 311

Rationale: If a person fails to respond to appropriate antimicrobial therapy and continues to be febrile for longer than 3 to 5 days, radiologic evaluation to rule out obstruction or renal abscess is indicated. Failure to do this can lead to spread of the infection to the perinephric space.

5. **What is the best management for xanthogranulomatous pyelonephritis?**

    a. Incision and drainage
    b. Percutaneous drainage
    c. Long-term antimicrobial therapy
    d. Nephrectomy
    e. Partial nephrectomy

Correct Answer: d   Reference Page: 331

Rationale: The best treatment is surgical removal of the kidney. Partial nephrectomy with removal of all the inflammatory mass is feasible but frozen section studies to rule out carcinoma may be difficult. If incision and drainage alone are performed rather than nephrectomy, the patient may continue to suffer from protracted debilitating illness and may develop a renal cutaneous fistula and an even more difficult nephrectomy will be necessary.

6. **Bacteriuria in the elderly should be treated if:**

a.   the patient is asymptomatic.
b.   the patient is symptomatic.
c.   infections are persistent.
d.   infections are recurrent.
e.   pyuria is present.

Correct Answer: b   Reference Page: 339
Rationale: Asymptomatic bacteriuria in the elderly is prevalent and unless urea-splitting organisms such as Proteus are present, no treatment is necessary. There is no evidence that prolonged asymptomatic bacteriuria significantly affects mortality in the elderly. If the patients are symptomatic, however, they should be treated.

7. **What is the most common cause of unresolved bacteriuria?**

a.   Bacteria resistant to the initial drug
b.   Azotemia
c.   Emergence of resistant strains
d.   Noncompliance
e.   Under dosage

Correct Answer: a   Reference Page: 305
Rationale: The most common cause of unresolved bacteriuria is initial natural resistance of the strain present in the urine. The second most common cause is emergence of strains which are marginally sensitive to the antimicrobial used to treat the patient's infection. In this setting subinhibitory concentrations of antimicrobials will be insufficient to kill all the bacteria present. The more resistant strains will survive and lead to and become the predominant strain. It is important therefore to prescribe medication that will exceed the minimal inhibitory concentration by the widest margin to be sure that the patient is compliant and takes the medications as directed.

8. **Catheter associated bacteriuria should be treated:**

a.   if pyuria occurs.
b.   if hematuria occurs.
c.   if the patient develops chills and a fever.
d.   as soon as the catheter is removed.
e.   when antimicrobial resistant bacteria are identified.

Correct Answer: c   Reference Page: 340

Rationale: Patients with indwelling catheters will develop bacteriuria at a rate of approximately 10% per day. Within 5 to 10 days, therefore, the majority of patients will have bacteriuria. If they are asymptomatic, the patients should not receive antimicrobial therapy because this will simply lead to development of resistant bacteria. On the other hand, if a patient becomes symptomatic with chills or fever then a culture should be performed and antimicrobial therapy instituted. Asymptomatic patients who are colonized with urea-splitting organisms should be treated until the bacteria are gone so that colonization with nonurea-splitting organisms can occur.

5
Urinary Tract Infections
Anthony J. Schaeffer

1. **What is the primary virulence factor for uropathogenic E. coli?**

    a.   Bacterial adherence
    b.   Hemolysin
    c.   Antigen
    d.   Lipopolysaccharide
    e.   Flagella

Correct Answer: a   Reference Page: 291

Rationale: It is well established that bacterial adherence to epithelial cells is an essential step in the initiation of urinary tract infections. If the bacteria cannot adhere then subsequent colonization and invasion will not occur. Bacteria adhere to specific binding sites in the urinary tract and their ability to adhere is associated with infection of the urethra, bladder, or kidney.

2. **The drug of choice for uncomplicated acute cystitis is:**

    a.   Nitrofurantoin.
    b.   TMP/SMX.
    c.   Cefallxin.
    d.   Noroxin.
    e.   Ampicillin.

Correct Answer: b   Reference Page: 304

Rationale: TMP-SMX offers the best spectrum of activity at the lowest cost. Noroxin is more effective but too expensive. Bacterial resistance to the other drugs is significantly higher than to TMP/SMX.

3. **What is the primary risk factor for recurrent urinary tract infections in women?**

    a.   Vaginal cell receptivity
    b.   Diaphragm use
    c.   Sexual intercourse
    d.   Increasing age
    e.   Menopausal status

Correct Answer: a   Reference Page: 295
Rationale: Adherence of bacteria to the vaginal mucosa with subsequent colonization is a critical step in ascending urinary tract infections. Women who are susceptible to infection have increased receptivity for bacteria and during periods of remission have a degree of receptivity for bacteria which approaches that of healthy women who are not colonized with bacteria and do not get urinary tract infections.

4.   **When should a woman who is on empiric antimicrobial therapy for acute pyelonephritis undergo radiologic evaluation?**

    a.   Immediately
    b.   If febrile for longer than 3 days
    c.   If there is a history of recurrent urinary tract infections
    d.   If blood cultures are positive
    e.   After the infection subsides

Correct Answer: b   Reference Page: 311
Rationale: If a person fails to respond to appropriate antimicrobial therapy and continues to be febrile for longer than 3 to 5 days, radiologic evaluation to rule out obstruction or renal abscess is indicated. Failure to do this can lead to spread of the infection to the perinephric space.

5.   **What is the best management for xanthogranulomatous pyelonephritis?**

    a.   Incision and drainage
    b.   Percutaneous drainage
    c.   Long-term antimicrobial therapy
    d.   Nephrectomy
    e.   Partial nephrectomy

Correct Answer: d   Reference Page: 331
Rationale: The best treatment is surgical removal of the kidney. Partial nephrectomy with removal of all the inflammatory mass is feasible but frozen section studies to rule out carcinoma may be difficult. If incision and drainage alone are performed rather than nephrectomy, the patient may continue to suffer from protracted debilitating illness and may develop a renal cutaneous fistula and an even more difficult nephrectomy will be necessary.

6. **Bacteriuria in the elderly should be treated if:**

    a. the patient is asymptomatic.
    b. the patient is symptomatic.
    c. infections are persistent.
    d. infections are recurrent.
    e. pyuria is present.

Correct Answer: b   Reference Page: 339

Rationale: Asymptomatic bacteriuria in the elderly is prevalent and unless urea-splitting organisms such as Proteus are present, no treatment is necessary. There is no evidence that prolonged asymptomatic bacteriuria significantly affects mortality in the elderly. If the patients are symptomatic, however, they should be treated.

7. **What is the most common cause of unresolved bacteriuria?**

    a. Bacteria resistant to the initial drug
    b. Azotemia
    c. Emergence of resistant strains
    d. Noncompliance
    e. Under dosage

Correct Answer: a   Reference Page: 305

Rationale: The most common cause of unresolved bacteriuria is initial natural resistance of the strain present in the urine. The second most common cause is emergence of strains which are marginally sensitive to the antimicrobial used to treat the patient's infection. In this setting subinhibitory concentrations of antimicrobials will be insufficient to kill all the bacteria present. The more resistant strains will survive and lead to and become the predominant strain. It is important therefore to prescribe medication that will exceed the minimal inhibitory concentration by the widest margin to be sure that the patient is compliant and takes the medications as directed.

8. **Catheter associated bacteriuria should be treated:**

    a. if pyuria occurs.
    b. if hematuria occurs.
    c. if the patient develops chills and a fever.
    d. as soon as the catheter is removed.
    e. when antimicrobial resistant bacteria are identified.

Correct Answer: c   Reference Page: 340

Rationale: Patients with indwelling catheters will develop bacteriuria at a rate of approximately 10% per day. Within 5 to 10 days, therefore, the majority of patients will have bacteriuria. If they are asymptomatic, the patients should not receive antimicrobial therapy because this will simply lead to development of resistant bacteria. On the other hand, if a patient becomes symptomatic with chills or fever then a culture should be performed and antimicrobial therapy instituted. Asymptomatic patients who are colonized with urea-splitting organisms should be treated until the bacteria are gone so that colonization with nonurea-splitting organisms can occur.

6
Management of Urologic Problems in Pregnancy
Jeffrey P. Weiss and Jay Y. Gillenwater

1. **A patient with a moderately symptomatic ureteral calculus during pregnancy is best treated by:**

   a. percutaneous nephrostomy.
   b. expectant observation and appropriate analgesics.
   c. placement of a ureteral stent.
   d. extracorporeal shock wave lithotripsy.
   e. open lithotomy.

   Correct Answer: b   Reference Page: 358
   Rationale: The majority of symptomatic stones during pregnancy will pass spontaneously; thus, the treatment of ureteral calculi during pregnancy is primarily expectant and the patient may be treated with any of the other techniques when pain is persistent or complications such as pyelonephritis or increasing hydronephrosis become problematic.

2. **Bacteriuria of pregnancy:**

   a. is defined as greater than 10,000 colony forming units per cc on a clean void specimen.
   b. directly results in prematurity, low birth rate and growth retardation.
   c. rarely progresses to pyelonephritis.
   d. causes fetal complications through its association with pyelonephritis.
   e. is usually associated with structural urinary defects.

   Correct Answer: d   Reference Page: 359
   Rationale: Because 20% to 40% of pregnant women with first trimester asymptomatic bacteriuria acquire pyelonephritis in the third trimester and because pyelonephritis of pregnancy is associated with low birth weight, growth retardation and premature labor, it is considered axiomatic that bacteriuria of pregnancy be both screened for and treated. Treatment may range from short courses of antibiotics with close follow-up or a single nightly dose of an antibiotic throughout the course of pregnancy.

3.   **Which one of the following antimicrobials is considered safe without reservation during pregnancy barring allergy?**

    a.   Penicillins
    b.   Sulfonamides
    c.   Trimethoprim-sulfa
    d.   Chloramphenicol
    e.   Tetracycline

Correct Answer: a   Reference Page: 355

Rationale: Sulfonamides are safe until 28 weeks gestation after which time there is a risk of fetal kernicterus in patients with glucose-6-phosphate dehydrogenase deficiency. Trimethoprim-sulfa is contraindicated because of possible teratogenicity and fetal folate antagonism. Chloramphenicol is contraindicated near term because of potential bone marrow depression and fetal gray syndrome. Tetracycline causes dysgenesis of fetal limbs and teeth.

4.   **Normal physiologic changes in the gravid state include which of the following?**

    a.   Decreased glomerular filtration rate
    b.   Sodium wasting
    c.   Hypercalciuria
    d.   Increased peripheral vascular resistance
    e.   Diminished levels of renin and angiotensin-II

Correct Answer: c   Reference Pages: 353-354

Rationale: Glomerular filtration rate (GFR) increases in pregnancy are primarily owing to increased cardiac output and decreased renal vascular resistance. Sodium homeostasis is maintained during pregnancy due to multiple offsetting factors: increase in GFR during pregnancy ordinarily would cause sodium loss due to the additional filtered load. Tubular reabsorption accounts for preservation of most of the sodium as does increased mineralocorticoid secretion; the antinatriuretic effect of estrogens is enhanced by induction of 21-hydroxylation of progesterone, yielding salt-retaining deoxycorticosterone. Hypercalciuria occurs primarily because of increased calcium filtration and excess intestinal calcium absorption secondary to high plasma levels of calcitriol. Peripheral vascular resistance is diminished during pregnancy in association with increased cardiac output. Renin and angiotensin-II levels increase during gestation owing to increases in prostaglandin E2 and prostacycline produced by the uterus, resulting in general vasodilation, decreased blood pressure and augmented vascular volume.

5.   **Roentgenographic imaging during pregnancy:**

  a.   is safe if limited to the third trimester.
  b.   may be done as a 2 or 3 "shot" urogram throughout pregnancy.
  c.   increases the fetal anomaly rate to 3%
  d.   is less accurate than sonography in diagnosis of acute urinary calculi.
  e.   delivers five rad to the fetus per abdominal film.

Correct Answer: b   Reference Page: 356
Rationale: Each abdominal film during pregnancy delivers only 0.2 rad to the fetus. Thus, two or three plain films taken in order to perform a satisfactory urogram provides a negligible exposure, well under the standard 1.5 rad for a standard urogram and far less than the 5 to 15 rad necessary to increase the risk of fetal anomalies to 3%. Urosonography is rarely helpful in diagnosis of acute urinary calculi because of the prevalence of physiologic hydronephrosis of pregnancy.

6.   **In comparing the two major causes of acute renal failure of pregnancy, acute tubular necrosis differs from renal cortical necrosis by virtue of which of the following?**

  a.   Acute tubular necrosis is clinically manifested by oligoanuric renal failure.
  b.   Renal cortical necrosis is associated with reversible renal failure.
  c.   Renal cortical necrosis occurs in a setting of disseminated intravascular coagulation.
  d.   Acute tubular necrosis results in renal cortical calcification once healing occurs.
  e.   Acute tubular necrosis results from progressive hydronephrosis of pregnancy.

Correct Answer: c   Reference Page: 361
Rationale: Acute tubular necrosis is associated with prerenal azotemia unlike renal cortical necrosis which occurs in a setting of disseminated intravascular coagulation, in turn caused by amniotic fluid embolism, abruptio placentae or intrauterine fetal demise. Transfusion reactions and sepsis may also predispose to renal cortical necrosis, for example, in a setting of chorioamnionitis, septic abortion and pyelonephritis. While acute tubular necrosis is associated with nonoliguric renal failure, renal cortical necrosis usually results in oligoanuric renal failure which progresses to chronic renal failure with renal cortical calcification. By contrast, acute tubular necrosis tends to resolve to normal renal function.

7
Urologic Laser Surgery
Douglas F. Milam and Joseph A. Smith, Jr.

1.   **Invasive squamous cell carcinoma of the penis is best treated for cure using:**

   a.   the CO2 laser
   b.   electrocoagulation
   c.   the Nd:YAG laser
   d.   the alexandrite laser
   e.   5-fluorouracil

Correct Answer: c   Reference Page: 373

Rationale: The Nd:YAG laser has been shown to be useful for curative therapy and organ preservation in properly selected patients with invasive squamous cell carcinoma of the penis. The carbon dioxide laser is useful for superficial lesions such as condylomata acuminata but does not produce a deep zone of coagulation which is necessary in patients with invasive carcinoma. Electrocoagulation produces an irregular area of tissue injury which is not useful for cancer treatment. The alexandrite laser was used to fragment ureteral and bladder stones. It is poorly absorbed by tissue and is not useful here. Five-fluorouracil has been shown to be active for superficial lesions such as Erythroplasia of Queyrat but is not useful for invasive cancer.

2.   **When treating penile condylomata, the CO2 laser should be set to produce _______ watt output.**

   a.   1
   b.   5
   c.   15
   d.   25
   e.   40

Correct Answer: b   Reference Page: 373

Rationale: CO2 laser energy is strongly absorbed by water. This produces strong tissue vaporization. Lower energy settings are used for skin ablation with the CO2 laser than are used for bladder and prostatic coagulation. One watt is generally insufficient for adequate tissue vaporization. Five watts is almost always sufficient, however. Fifteen, 25 and 40 watts exposure would produce rapid tissue vaporization creating a tissue ablator.

3.   **Laser prostatectomy produces results similar to TURP in which of the following objective measures?**

   a.   Peak urinary flow rate (Qmax)
   b.   Mean urinary flow rate (Q)
   c.   American Urological Association Symptom Score
   d.   Incidence of bladder neck contracture
   e.   Incidence of blood transfusion

Correct Answer: c   Reference Pages: 385-386
Rationale: Several studies have demonstrated similar decreases in the American Urologic Association symptom score following Nd:YAG coagulation laser prostatectomy and transurethral resection of the prostate. These same studies have indicated that the urinary flow rate improved substantially following laser prostatectomy but only about two-thirds as much as TURP. Bladder neck contracture and blood transfusion are rare complications of laser prostatectomy, occurring much less frequently than following TURP.

4.   **Which parameter influences the interaction of laser light with tissue?**

   a.   Tissue color
   b.   Power density
   c.   Wavelength
   d.   Presence of carbon
   e.   All of above

Correct Answer: e   Reference Pages: 370-371
Rationale: Tissue color is an important determinate of which wavelengths of incident light is absorbed or reflected. Likewise, the laser wavelength determines the depth of coagulation or extent of vaporization depending upon the intensity of tissue absorption of various wavelengths. Power density is important since very high power exposures change tissue absorption characteristics. High power density exposure can produce tissue carbonization. Carbon black is a strong absorber of almost all wavelengths. Extensive surface carbonization can prevent incident laser light from reaching deeper tissues.

5.   **The principle advantage of Nd:YAG photocoagulation over TURBT for the treatment of superficial bladder tumor is:**

   a.   decreased rate of recurrence.
   b.   decreased intraoperative cost.
   c.   decreased morbidity (outpatient surgery).
   d.   decreased operative time.
   e.   need for local anesthesia only.

Correct Answer: c   Reference Page: 376

Rationale: Nd:YAG photocoagulation for superficial bladder tumors has a significantly decreased morbidity compared to routine TURBT. Bladder perforation does not occur and even extensive tumors can usually be treated on an outpatient basis. Delayed bowel perforation is a rare complication which can be prevented by modification of the treatment technique. Nd:YAG photocoagulation does not appear to decrease the rate of recurrence compared to TURBT. The intraoperative cost is equivalent or slightly greater than TURBT and the operative time is also similar. Superficial bladder tumors of substantial size require regional or general anesthesia when treated with both the Nd:YAG laser or TURBT.

6. **The best laser source for coagulation laser prostatectomy in a noncontact mode is:**

a. KTP (Potassium Titanyl Phosphate)
b. Nd:YAG (Neodymium: Yttrium, Aluminium, Garnet)
c. Holmium
d. Alexandrite
e. Diode laser 615 nm

Correct Answer: b   Reference Pages: 380-381, 387

Rationale: The 1064 nm wavelength of the continuous wave Nd:YAG laser has a nearly optimal degree of absorption. This allows for deep tissue coagulation in a non-contact mode. The KTP laser is useful for vaporization prostatectomy or vaporization transurethral incision of the prostate. However, the coagulation defect produced is too superficial to be used in the conventional non-contact side-firing coagulation mode. The holmium laser has been used for prostatic ablation. This laser source is incompatible with most side-firing laser prostatectomy devices, however. The alexandrite laser is not useful for side-firing non-contact laser prostatectomy. The same is true for diode lasers operating at 615 nm wavelengths. This wavelength of laser may be useful for interstitial prostatic thermotherapy, though. Diode lasers operating between 800 and 1100 nm are useful for side-firing non-contact prostatectomy.

8
Malignancy: Underlying Concepts of
Natural History, Etiology, and Treatment
William C. DeWolf

1.   **The basic principles governing our understanding of cancer are:**

    a.   based on abnormal transduction of "signals" through the cell membrane secondary to oncogene function.

    b.   related to factors governing loss of cellular senescence, or normal number of "population doublings."

    c.   twofold: a) cancer is a disease of genetic malfunction and b) there must be more than one mistake for cancer to occur.

    d.   related to loss of "stabilizing factors" for cellular function such as provided by "suppressor genes."

    e.   involved with abnormal cell cycle regulation.

Correct Answer: c   Reference Page: 395

2.   **Oncogenes represent altered forms of normally occurring protooncogenes. These alterations are best characterized as:**

    a.   always associated with mutations.

    b.   alteration by either gene dosage (amplification) or alteration in function by change in structure (mutation).

    c.   affecting transmission of signals through the cell membrane.

    d.   stimulating phosphorylation.

    e.   a necessary requirement for malignant transformation.

Correct Answer: b   Reference Page: 414, table 8-5

3.   **One major class of cancer associated genes are the tumor suppressor genes. They differ from oncogenes in that:**

    a.   mutations can occur sporadically.

    b.   mutations in such genes can be inherited.

    c.   they affect signal transduction.

    d.   they affect a narrow range of tumors.

    e.   they affect growth stimulating cellular properties.

Correct Answer: b   Reference Page: 415

4.   **A unique feature of the ureterosigmoidostomy anastomosis is that cancers occur at the suture line in at least 1 of 10 patients followed long term. The etiology:**

a.   is unknown but may be related to an interaction between scarring and carcinogens because tumors occur principally along the suture line.

b.   is known and related to nitrosourea activation of the H ras protooncogene by guanine to adenine transition mutations.

c.   relates to the occurrence of transitional cell cancers through the production of ornithine decarboxylase which may induce polyamines that act as a promoter in the malignant transformation of colonic tissue.

d.   applies only to ureterosigmoidostomies and not to other types of manipulations juxtaposing transitional epithelium to intestinal epithelium.

e.   occurs only when urine is actively passing over the anastomosis.

Correct Answer: a   Reference Page: 424

5.   **It is commonly known that chronic urothelial irritation by urinary calculi can be associated with malignant transformation. The principal behind this association is:**

a.   chronic inflammation inactivates tumor suppressor genes.

b.   the irritation by a stone induces a "genotoxic" event resulting in a mutuation.

c.   the implantation of various irritant substances into the bladder leads to malignancy through a "nongenotoxic" event resulting in cancer with increasing time of exposure.

d.   the stone acts as an "initiator" in the cascade of events leading to malignancy.

e.   tumors grow by a process of clonal evolution driven by mutation.

Correct Answer: c   Reference Page: 429

6.   **The major histocompatibility (MHC) antigens:**

a.   are teleologically present to prevent tissue from being transplanted from one organism to another.

b.   are of three basic types.

c.   are present to deliver and present "foreign antigens" to the immune system.

d.   help explain why nude mice (without T cells) do not have a higher incidence of spontaneous tumors than normal mice.

e.   are the "targets" for NK cells.

Correct Answer: c   Reference Page: 431

7.   **Apoptosis, or programmed cell death:**

a.   is an important phenomenon that, in normal circumstances, leads to an imbalance between cell renewal and cell death.
b.   occurs very late on the evolutionary tree and involves only mammals.
c.   is an organized energy dependent process similar to necrotic cell death.
d.   is important to conceptually understand cancer therapy because many treatment forms including radiation and chemotherapy involve induction of apoptosis in some tumors.
e.   is a multigenic process with defined and known steps that initiate the process.

Correct Answer: d   Reference Page: 439

9
Calculus Formation
Alan D. Jenkins

1. **Nephrocalcin is an acidic glycoprotein that:**

   a. promotes polymerization of matrix.
   b. catalyzes the degradation of PTH.
   c. inhibits calcium oxalate crystal growth.
   d. gamma carboxylates glutamic acid residues.
   e. promotes calcium oxalate crystal growth.

   Correct Answer: c   Reference Page: 464
   Rationale: Nephrocalcin is a high molecular weight inhibitor of calcium oxalate crystal growth and aggregation. Some patients with calcium oxalate stone disease have an abnormal nephrocalcin in which many of the glutamic acid residues do not have gamma carboxyl groups. The gamma carboxyglutamic acid residues of normal nephrocalcin avidly bind calcium.

2. **Oral citrate can be an effective treatment for idiopathic calcium urolithiasis because it:**

   a. is rapidly absorbed in the jejunum and excreted unchanged in the urine.
   b. binds urinary calcium and decreases calcium oxalate supersaturation.
   c. increases the urinary concentration of crystal aggregation inhibitors.
   d. increases the urinary concentration of low molecular weight inhibitors.
   e. increases the urinary concentration of crystal growth inhibitors.

   Correct Answer: b   Reference Page: 464
   Rationale: After gastrointestinal absorption, citrate passes through the liver where it is metabolized to bicarbonate. The alkalinizing effect of citrate decreases renal reabsorption of citrate and increases urinary excretion. The major effect of citrate is achieved through complexation of calcium and reduction of calcium oxalate supersaturation.

3. **A 54-year-old woman has a 30-year history of recurrent calcium oxalate stone formation. She has had several surgical procedures for the complications of Crohn's disease. A 24-hour urine likely will reveal:**

   a. low volume, high citrate, high oxalate.
   b. high volume, low citrate, high oxalate.
   c. low volume, low citrate, low oxalate.

    d.   high volume, low citrate, high oxalate.
    e.   low volume, low citrate, high oxalate.

Correct Answer: e   Reference Page: 477
Rationale: This patient has enteric hyperoxaluria in which the basic defect is intestinal malabsorption of bile acids, fats, and electrolytes. The malabsorbed fats bind calcium, thereby increasing the amount of free oxalate available for absorption. Malabsorption of fluids and electrolytes leads to a reduced urine volume, intracellular acidosis, and low urinary citrate excretion.

4.   **A 29-year-old fashion model passes a ureteral calculus composed of ammonium acid urate. A 24-hour urine volume is 973 ml. The sample contains little sodium, potassium, or citrate. This patient should be treated with:**

    a.   withdrawal of her laxatives.
    b.   slow release potassium citrate.
    c.   a liquid preparation of sodium citrate.
    d.   fluids and allopurinol.
    e.   sodium bicarbonate and acetazolamide.

Correct Answer: a   Reference Page: 480
Rationale: Ammonium acid urate stone formation has been reported in women with a history of laxative abuse. GI loss of fluid and electrolytes leads to extracellular volume depletion and intracellular acidosis. Urine volume and the excretion of sodium, potassium, and citrate fall. All of the listed therapies would help, but withdrawal of the laxatives is the only choice that would reverse the underlying pathophysiology.

5.   **The adverse metabolic effects of primary hyperoxaluria can be corrected with:**

    a.   pyridoxine.
    b.   liver transplantation.
    c.   potassium citrate.
    d.   renal transplantation.
    e.   orthophosphate.

Correct Answer: b   Reference Page: 439
Rationale: Enzyme deficiencies are responsible for both types of primary hyperoxaluria. A few investigators have reported reversal of the metabolic defect and the complications of primary hyperoxaluria after liver transplantation or combined liver-kidney transplantation. Pyridoxine, orthophosphate, and potassium citrate can be used to treat primary hyperoxaluria, but these drugs do not affect the enzymatic disorder.

10
Perioperative Care
W. Scott McDougal

1. **The first sign of the water intoxication syndrome during a TURP is:**

   a.   rise in blood pressure.
   b.   bradycardia.
   c.   tachypnea.
   d.   elevated CVP.
   e.   changes in sensorium.

   Correct Answer: d   Reference Page: 523
   Rationale: The first change which occurs is a rising CVP or a left atrial pressure. The other signs listed occur but generally later in the course of the disease.

2. **When glycine is used as the irrigant during a TURP:**

   a.   water intoxication does not occur.
   b.   ammonium intoxication may occur.
   c.   hemolysis occurs with rapid absorption.
   d.   visualization is improved as compared to water.
   e.   hyperkalemia may occur.

   Correct Answer: b   Reference Page: 523
   Rationale: Ammonium intoxication may be a complication as glycine is metabolized systemically. Because the irrigant is isosmotic, hemolysis is limited and hyperkalemia is generally not a complication. Moreover, because of this, visualization is not as good as when water is used. Since water intoxication is dependent on fluid overload and dilutional hyponatremia there is the same frequency of this syndrome irrespective of whether water or glycine is used as the irrigant.

3. **When urinary intestinal diversion using ileum results in a hyperchloremic metabolic acidosis the primary mechanism responsible is:**

   a.   ammonium transport.
   b.   ammonia transport.
   c.   bicarbonate loss.
   d.   chloride absorption.
   e.   proton absorption.

Correct Answer: a   Reference Page: 525

Rationale: The primary mechanism of the hyperchloremic metabolic acidosis of urinary intestinal diversion is ammonium absorption in exchange for a proton. In conjunction with this, the chloride bicarbonate exchanger results in chloride absorption with bicarbonate secretion. The net effect is ammonium chloride absorption in exchange for carbonic acid.

4.   **A mechanical bowel prep results in:**

a.   a more rapid return of bowel function postoperatively.
b.   a reduction in the number of bacteria per cc of fecal material.
c.   a higher incidence of pseudomembranous enterocolitis.
d.   increased tumor implantation on the suture line.
e.   a reduction in total number of bacteria present in the bowel.

Correct Answer: e   Reference Page: 527

Rationale: A mechanical bowel prep reduces the total number of bacteria in the bowel, but not the concentration per cc of feces. The rest of the complications listed result when antibiotics are added to the regimen.

5.   **The risk of a pulmonary embolism is best prevented by:**

a.   beginning the prophylaxis prior to induction of anesthesia.
b.   minidose heparin.
c.   coumadin begun postoperatively.
d.   pneumatic compression stockings.
e.   early ambulation.

Correct Answer: a   Reference Page: 533

Rationale: Whatever the prophylaxis, it is most effective when begun preoperatively prior to the induction of anesthesia.

Renal Injuries

Jack W. McAninch

1. **Gross hematuria is noted after urethral catheterization following blunt abdominal trauma. This finding suggests:**

   a. renal contusion.
   b. bladder rupture.
   c. renal parenchymal laceration.
   d. major renal vascular injury.
   e. any of the above.

   Correct Answer: e   Reference Page: 541

   Rationale: The degree (gross or microscopic) does not correlate with the degree of renal injury. Gross hematuria is present in a high percentage (> 95%) of bladder ruptures. Renal imaging and cystoscopy would be required in this patient.

2. **The diagnostic study to best demonstrate a parenchymal laceration, urinary extravasation and the extent of the retroperitoneal hematoma is:**

   a. excretory urogram.
   b. abdominal computed tomography.
   c. nephrotomography.
   d. arteriography.
   e. magnetic resonance imaging.

   Correct Answer: b   Reference Page: 543-544

   Rationale: Computed tomography is the only study listed that provides the information requested on the proposed injury: parenchymal laceration, urinary extravasation and the extent of the retroperitoneal hematoma.

3. **Renal imaging is *not* necessary following blunt abdominal trauma in a(n):**

   a. ten-year-old child with microscopic hematuria.
   b. adult with gross hematuria.
   c. adult with microscopic hematuria and SBP < 90 mmHg.
   d. adult with microscopic hematuria and SBP of 100/80.
   e. a deceleration injury with no hematuria.

Correct Answer: c   Reference Pages: 541-542

Rationale: Emerging data provide strong evidence that adult patients sustaining blunt trauma who do not have hypotension (SBP < 90 mmHg) can be followed safely clinically without performing imaging. All other patients listed should have imaging studies.

4.   **Renal exploration should be performed when a known renal injury exists in the following circumstance:**

    a.   abdominal exploration is being done by the general surgeon.
    b.   persistent renal bleeding is noted.
    c.   the CT shows a major parenchymal laceration.
    d.   urinary extravasation is noted.
    e.   a renal stab wound.

Correct Answer: b   Reference Page: 546

Rationale: Persistent bleeding from a renal injury is an absolute indication for renal exploration. All the other possibilities are not absolute indications for exploration.

5.   **The primary abnormality noted in acute renal artery thrombosis caused by blunt deceleration injury is:**

    a.   intimal arterial tear.
    b.   arterial adventitial contusion.
    c.   shock with poor renal arterial perfusion.
    d.   primary injury to the arterial muscularis.
    e.   severe renal contusion resulting in poor venous drainage.

Correct Answer: a   Reference Page: 547

Rationale: The intima of the renal artery has little elasticity, and excessive stretch, during deceleration injury can result in intimal disruption which causes thrombus development.

6.   **The characteristic of a gunshot injury which provides the most information regarding tissue damage is:**

    a.   location of the entrance wound.
    b.   distance from which the weapon was fired.
    c.   mass of the bullet.
    d.   velocity of the bullet.
    e.   bullet fragmentation.

Correct Answer: d   Reference Page: 541

Rationale: The velocity of the bullet is the most important factor directly related to the tissue damage and the kinetic energy expended for a gunshot wound.

7.   **The most common cause of arteriovenous fistula formation following renal trauma is:**

   a.   deceleration injury.
   b.   gunshot wound.
   c.   stab wound.
   d.   attempted renal laceration repair.
   e.   mass ligation of the renal artery and vein at the time of nephrectomy.

Correct Answer: c   Reference Page: 552

Rationale: Stab wounds, not surgically repaired, result in the highest incidence of arteriovenous fistulas in the postinjury period.

11B
Ureteral Injuries
Joseph N. Corriere, Jr.

1. **During an abdominal hysterectomy, the lower third of the right ureter is ligated. After deligation the ureter looks contused but has peristalsis. The next step is:**

    a. close the wound.
    b. place a ureteral stent.
    c. wrap the ureter in omentum.
    d. resect the segment and perform a ureteroureterostomy.
    e. perform a ureteroneocystostomy.

    Correct Answer: b   Reference Page: 559

    Rationale: This is basically a crush injury. However, the blood supply is intact as documented by the good peristalsis. In that setting, placing a stent is quite reasonable. If there is any concern whatsoever about the blood supply, then a reimplantation should be performed. An injury in the lower third of the ureter should never be repaired with a ureteroureterostomy since a ureteroneocystostomy has a much higher success rate. Wrapping the ureter in omentum or closing the wound has a higher risk of more permanent injury.

2. **Three weeks after an abdominal hysterectomy an IVP done because of left flank pain reveals an obstructed ureter at the level of the iliac vessels. An attempt to pass a retrograde stent fails. The next step is:**

    a. repeat the IVP in one month.
    b. place a percutaneous nephrostomy and antegrade stent.
    c. perform a ureteroureterostomy.
    d. perform a ureteroneocystostomy.
    e. perform a transureteroureterostomy.

    Correct Answer: b   Reference Page: 560

    Rationale: If a stent can be passed, this will usually solve the problem if the ureter was tied with an absorbable material. If not, of course, repair is indicated. Repeating an IVP in a month would be inadvisable because further damage from the obstruction could occur, and open surgery usually, but not always, can be avoided. Meanwhile, the indwelling stent will relieve the hydronephrosis.

3. **Two months after an abdominal hysterectomy, a patient is found to have a left hydronephrosis and a lower left ureterovaginal fistula. A percutaneous antegrade stent is passed by the fistula site into the bladder. The next step is:**

a. observation.
b. perform a ureteroureterostomy.
c. perform a ureteroneocystostomy.
d. perform a transureteroureterostomy.
e. perform a balloon dilatation and incision of the fistula site.

Correct Answer: a   Reference Page: 560
Rationale: In this setting, the ureter will usually heal over the stent and surgery is not necessary. Balloon dilatation could increase the size of the fistula and further injure the ureter.

12
Trauma to the Lower Urinary Tract
Joseph N. Corriere, Jr.

1. **The hallmark diagnostic sign that a patient with a pelvic fracture has an injury to the urinary bladder is:**

    a. hematuria.
    b. dysuria.
    c. urinary frequency.
    d. lower abdominal pain.
    e. hypotension.

    Correct Answer: a   Reference Page: 564
    Rationale: Every patient with an injury to the bladder has hematuria and it is almost always gross hematuria.

2. **Definitive diagnosis of a ruptured bladder is made by performing a(n):**

    a. IVP.
    b. ultrasound of the abdomen.
    c. CT of the abdomen.
    d. static cystogram.
    e. VCU.

    Correct Answer: d   Reference Page: 564
    Rationale: Only a static cystogram with the bladder filled in the retrograde fashion (forcibly distended) to 250–300cc will definitely diagnose a ruptured bladder. Many times the cystogram on an IVP or CT scan using intravenous contrast will not demonstrate extravasation even though the bladder is ruptured..

3. **Appropriate therapy for an intraperitoneal bladder rupture from external violence in a man is:**

    a. 10 days of Foley catheter drainage.
    b. 10 days of percutaneous suprapubic catheter drainage.
    c. 10 days of formal suprapubic catheter drainage.
    d. percutaneous perivesical drainage and catheter placement.
    e. formal surgical repair and catheter drainage.

Correct Answer: e   Reference Page: 568
Rationale: After an intraperitoneal bladder rupture urine usually preferentially leaks into the peritoneal cavity, even with catheter drainage. All patients must have formal repair to prevent peritonitis.

4.   **Extraperitoneal rupture of the urinary bladder that extends into the bladder neck in a child is best treated by:**

   a.   10 days of Foley catheter drainage.
   b.   10 days of percutaneous SP tube drainage.
   c.   10 days of formal SP tube drainage.
   d.   percutaneous perivesical drainage and catheter placement.
   e.   formal surgical repair and catheter drainage.

Correct Answer: e   Reference Page: 569
Rationale: If formal repair of a bladder neck injury is not performed, incontinence or bladder neck contracture may occur.

5.   **Blood at the urethral meatus in a patient with a fractured pelvis portends a(n):**

   a.   intraperitoneal bladder rupture.
   b.   extraperitoneal bladder rupture.
   c.   rupture of the posterior urethra.
   d.   rupture of the anterior urethra.
   e.   fracture of the penis.

Correct Answer: c   Reference Page: 570
Rationale: Posterior urethral rupture associated with a pelvic fracture usually results in blood leaking from the injury out the urethral meatus.

6.   **The diagnosis of a ruptured urethra is best made by:**

   a.   urethral catheterization.
   b.   cystoscopy.
   c.   VCU.
   d.   retrograde urethrogram.
   e.   ultrasound.

Correct Answer: d   Reference Page: 570
Rationale: Only the overdistended urethra using contrast can delineate if an injury has occurred as well as the extent of the damage and type of injury. Instrumentation of any type must be avoided or the injury may be made worse.

7. **Patients with a complete anterior urethral rupture with extensive perineal hematoma formation are best treated by:**

    a.   urethral catheterization and observation.
    b.   suprapubic tube placement and delayed repair.
    c.   endoscopic realignment.
    d.   immediate debridement and repair.
    e.   suprapubic tube placement, hematoma drainage and repair.

Correct Answer: b   Reference Page: 579

Rationale: Conservative therapy by urinary diversion and observation will allow the hematoma to resolve and the injury to declare itself. Early aggressive instrumentation will result in extensive removal of contused tissue thought to be necrotic. If left alone to recover it will heal.

13
The Adrenals
Andrew C. Novick and Stuart S. Howards

1. **The most common cause of Cushing's syndrome is:**

   a. adrenal adenoma.
   b. adrenal carcinoma.
   c. Cushing's disease.
   d. exogenous glucocorticoids.
   e. ectopic ACTH secretion.

   Correct Answer: d   Reference Page: 594
   Rationale: The most common cause of Cushing's syndrome is exogenously administered glucocorticoids. The most common cause of endogenous Cushing's syndrome is excessive ACTH secretion from the pituitary gland (Cushing's disease) which accounts for 75% of such cases.

2. **The highest plasma ACTH levels are observed in:**

   a. Cushing's disease.
   b. ectopic ACTH secretion.
   c. adrenal adenoma.
   d. adrenal carcinoma.
   e. primary adrenal hyperplasia.

   Correct Answer: b   Reference Page: 596
   Rationale: Patients with ectopic secretion of ACTH demonstrate the highest plasma ACTH levels, usually in the range of 200 to 1000 pg/ml. Plasma ACTH levels are also elevated in Cushing's disease but not to the same extent (40 to 100 pg/ml). Plasma ACTH levels are reduced in patients with adrenal adenoma, adrenal carcinoma, or primary adrenal hyperplasia.

3. **The primary treatment for Cushing's disease is:**

   a. bilateral adrenalectomy.
   b. transsphenoidal hypophysectomy.
   c. pituitary irradiation.
   d. mitotane (op-DDD).
   e. cyproheptadine.

Correct Answer: b   Reference Page 598

Rationale: Transsphenoidal hypophysectomy is the treatment of choice for Cushing's disease, and the success rate varies from 70% to 95%. This treatment is less morbid than bilateral adrenalectomy and avoids the complication of Nelson's syndrome. Pituitary irradiation has only a 20% cure rate in adults. Bilateral adrenalectomy is reserved for patients who have failed pituitary surgery.

4.   **The most accurate diagnostic test for primary aldosteronism is:**

    a.   serum potassium < 3.0 meq/1.
    b.   elevated serum aldosterone that is suppressed after saline infusion.
    c.   elevated serum aldosterone that is not suppressed after saline infusion.
    d.   low plasma renin activity.
    e.   elevated urinary aldosterone level.

Correct Answer: c   Reference Page: 599

Rationale: The most accurate diagnostic test for establishing the biochemical diagnosis of primary aldosteronism is the demonstration of elevated serum or urinary aldosterone levels, and the failure of such elevated levels to suppress following salt loading. Hypokalemia and hyporeninemia are less specific findings.

5.   **The most accurate technique for localizing an aldosterone-producing adrenal cortical adenoma is:**

    a.   adrenal venography.
    b.   adrenal venous aldosterone measurements.
    c.   CT scan.
    d.   MRI scan.
    e.   MIBG scan.

Correct Answer: b   Reference Page: 600

Rationale: Adrenal vein catheterization with sampling and analysis of the effluent for aldosterone is the most precise way to localize an aldosteronoma. Since it is an invasive study, a CT or MRI scan is usually obtained first. Adrenal venous sampling is reserved for patients with a biochemical diagnosis of aldosteronism and negative noninvasive imaging studies.

6.   **Malignant pheochromocytomas produce more norepinephrine due to a deficiency of:**

    a.   monoamine oxidase.
    b.   tyrosine hydroxylase.
    c.   phenylethanolamine N-methyltransferase.

d.   1-aromatic amino acid decarboxylase.
e.   phenylalanine hydroxylase.

Correct Answer: c   Reference Page: 603
Rationale: Extraadrenal and malignant pheochromocytomas produce more norephinephrine and less epinephrine than benign adrenal pheochromocytomas due to a deficiency of phenylethanolamine N-methyltransferase in the former. This enzyme promotes the conversion of norephinephrine to epinephrine in sympathetic tissue.

7.   **The preferred surgical approach for removal of a solitary 3.5 cm left adrenal pheochromocytoma is:**

a.   midline transabdominal.
b.   subcostal transabdominal.
c.   thoracoabdominal.
d.   extraperitoneal flank.
e.   posterior lumbotomy.

Correct Answer: d   Reference Page: 604
Rationale: With the availability of improved localization techniques, it is no longer routinely necessary to explore the abdomen in patients with pheochromocytoma. Therefore, in selected patients with a small adrenal tumor and no evidence of extraadrenal disease or multiple tumors, a unilateral extraperitoneal surgical approach may be used.

14
The Kidney
W. Scott McDougal

1. **The glomerular filtration rate is best determined using a substance which is:**

   a. secreted by the proximal tubule.
   b. reabsorbed by the proximal tubule.
   c. neither secreted nor reabsorbed by the tubule.
   d. secreted and reabsorbed by the tubule.
   e. a sugar.

   Correct Answer: c   Reference Page: 619
   Rationale: The best substance to measure glomerular filtration is one which is freely filtered by the glomerulus and neither secreted nor reabsorbed by the tubule. Insulin, a sugar is the gold standard.

2. **In the proximal tubule:**

   a. 80% of the filtrate is reabsorbed.
   b. glucose is secreted.
   c. urinary acidification occurs.
   d. potassium is secreted.
   e. fluid is concentrated.

   Correct Answer: a   Reference Page: 620
   Rationale: In the proximal tubule 80% to 90% of filtrate is reabsorbed isosmotically. This portion of the nephron is exceedingly active in glucose, amino acid and electrolyte reabsorption. Acidification and potassium secretion occur in the distal tubule.

3. **Determining glomerular filtration in patients with urinary intestinal diversion requires:**

   a. the use of insulin.
   b. is most accurately performed by radionuclide scan.
   c. must be done under diuretic conditions.
   d. is best performed using serum decay methods.
   e. cannot be performed accurately.

Correct Answer: c   Reference Page: 627

Rationale: Because the intestinal epithelium reabsorbs solute excreted by the kidney, this must be minimized in order to accurately measure glomerular filtration rate. This may be accomplished by establishing a diuresis which reduces the time of exposure and the concentration to the intestinal epithelium.

4.   **Initial management of hyperkalemia in patients with acute renal failure involves:**

    a.   intravenous sodium bicarbonate.
    b.   intravenous glucose and insulin.
    c.   PO ion exchange resin.
    d.   intravenous calcium gluconate.
    e.   dialysis.

Correct Answer: a   Reference Page: 629

Rationale: All of the above are used to reduce serum potassium. However, initially correcting the acidosis with sodium bicarbonate and if necessary, stabilizing the myocardium with calcium gluconate are preferred. If this does not correct the situation and the hyperkalemia is life threatening glucose and insulin may be employed. In order to permanently lower the potassium the use of ion exchange resins and/or dialysis is instituted subsequently.

5.   **Radiocontrast renal failure is most likely to occur in a patient with:**

    a.   compromised renal function.
    b.   diabetes mellitus.
    c.   dehydration.
    d.   multiple myeloma.
    e.   advanced age.

Correct Answer: a   Reference Page: 634

Rationale: Although all of the above add to the risk of developing contrast nephropathy, the most significant is compromised renal function, particularly in a patient who is already unstable, either due to trauma with vascular instability or metabolic instability due to such diseases as diabetes.

15
Renal, Perirenal, and Ureteral Neoplasms
Scott B. Jennings and W. Marston Linehan

1.   Mutations of the VHL gene are seen in the following renal tumors:

a.   renal cell carcinomas associated with von Hippel-Lindau disease.
b.   sporadic clear cell renal carcinomas.
c.   papillary renal cell carcinomas.
d.   a and b only.
e.   a, b, and c

Correct Answer: d   Reference Page: 653
Rationale: Tumor suppressor genes are thought to be implicated in the pathogenesis of many human neoplasms. However, direct evidence has been shown in only a few tumor types. Identification of the VHL gene is an example of the increasing molecular genetic sophistication currently being applied in urological research. Elucidation of the mechanism of action of the VHL gene and its product protein should provide new avenues for diagnosis and treatment of most renal cell carcinomas.

2.   Many patients with benign renal tumors undergo nephrectomy because:

a.   renal masses frequently cause symptoms and require treatment.
b.   clinical features to distinguish benign from malignant renal tumors are lacking.
c.   benign renal tumors are extremely rare.
d.   many benign renal tumors progress to become malignant.
e.   nephrectomy is the only effective treatment.

Correct Answer: b   Reference Page: 646
Rationale: As more and more small asymptomatic renal masses are discovered by ultrasound and CT, there will inevitably be an increased number of benign renal masses removed by urologists. At this time, clinical, radiological, and pathological features based on partial tumor sampling (i.e., needle biopsy) may be misleading, and thus the only sure diagnosis is provided by complete removal of the tumor, which has traditionally included total nephrectomy. However, there is an increasing body of evidence to support the role of partial nephrectomy for small renal cancers, and this option should also be considered.

3.   The most important prognostic indicator in patients with renal cell carcinoma is:

a. tumor stage.
b. tumor grade.
c. tumor size.
d. absence of vena caval involvement.
e. all of the above.

Correct Answer: a   Reference Page: 660

Rationale: Although many factors have been examined, tumor stage at the time of surgical exploration is the most powerful known prognostic indicator. Ultimately, tumor stage may prove to be as important as or more important than extent of surgical resection (as long as all tumor is removed), but this premise has not yet been examined by randomized trials.

4. **Which statement regarding immunotherapy for metastatic renal cell carcinoma is false?**

    a. High-dose intravenous interleukin-2 is the only FDA-approved agent for treatment of patients with metastatic renal cell carcinoma.
    b. Overall response rates of 15% to 20% are seen in most series of patients treated with various immunotherapeutic agents.
    c. Addition of α-interferon, LAK cells, or TIL to interleukin-2 has not been shown to be more effective than interleukin-2 alone.
    d. High dose intravenous interleukin-2 is more effective than low-dose intravenous or subcutaneous administration.
    e. Interleukin-2 appears to produce more durable responses than α-interferon.

Correct Answer: d   Reference Page: 668

Rationale: Although immunotherapy appears to more effective than other systemic therapies in patients with metastatic renal cell carcinoma, many questions remain regarding choice of agent, dosage, routes of administration, and combination therapy. Surprisingly few randomized trials have been performed to guide clinicians in their choice of therapy for these patients. For the moment, high-dose intravenous interleukin-2 appears to be the most efficacious agent, but it is hoped that clinical trials currently underway will clarify some of these issues.

5. **Etiologic factors implicated in the pathogenesis of both renal cell carcinomas and transitional cell carcinomas of the renal pelvis and ureter include:**

    a. diuretic use.
    b. obesity.
    c. asbestos exposure.
    d. formaldehyde fumes.
    e. cigarette smoking.

Correct Answer: d   Reference Pages: 651, 669

Rationale: Although many agents and etiologic factors have bene evaluated, cigarette smoking is the only major risk factor identified to date which seems to be important in the development of both renal cell carcinoma and transitional cell carcinoma (and other malignancies). Most other etiologic factors seem to convey only a mild increased risk, and their relative importance is unclear.

6. **Conservative treatment of some patients with transitional cell carcinoma of the renal pelvis or ureter is effective because:**

   a. urothelial tumors are usually unifocal.
   b. recurrence rates following conservative therapy are quite low.
   c. tumor grade and stage are more important than extent of surgical resection.
   d. the high risk of contralateral disease makes preservation of renal function imperative.
   e. low-grade tumors can be accurately diagnosed prior to surgery.

Correct Answer: c   Reference Page: 674

Rationale: Although patients with low-grade and low-stage tumors do well following conservative therapy, it can be very difficult to prospectively identify these patients because of the inherent diagnostic uncertainties associated with urothelial tumors. Radical nephroureterectomy remains the treatment of choice for most patients, and obviates the problems of tumor multifocality and local recurrence. However, conservative therapy clearly can play a role in the management of some patients.

7. **In the evaluation of suspected renal masses:**

   a. MRI is more expensive but offers no real advantage over CT.
   b. advantages of CT scanning over angiography include greater sensitivity and more accurate staging.
   c. most masses on IVP prove to be solid tumors.
   d. a mass seen on IVP but not on ultrasound is pathognomic for a hypertrophied column of Bertin.
   e. percutaneous aspiration of cysts is often necessary to confirm the diagnosis.

Correct Answer: b   Reference Page: 643

Rationale: Although multiple modalities are available for evaluation of renal masses, CT scanning with and without contrast is the most valuable single test, and in many cases is the only test needed to diagnose and stage a renal mass. However, each of the other modalities is commonly used, and in some cases all available methods must be used. Urologists should be familiar with the relative strengths and weaknesses of each modality and should develop a systematic approach to the evaluation of renal masses.

16
Stone Treatment
J. Patrick Spirnak and Martin I. Resnick

1.   **All of the following statements regarding renal anatomy are true *except*:**

   a.   Based on the segmental artery distribution, there are four surgical segments of the kidney.
   b.   Collateral circulation is absent between the segmental arteries.
   c.   In over 50% of kidneys, the anterior branch is the first branch off the renal artery.
   d.   The polar calyces are often single, whereas the remainder of the calyces are paired.
   e.   There is an avascular plane between the anterior and posterior segments of the kidney.

Correct Answer: c   Reference Pages: 698-700
Rationale: In over 50% of the kidneys, the posterior branch is the first branch off the renal artery.

2.   **All of the following statements regarding kidney stone surgery are true *except*:**

   a.   During a posterior lumbotomy approach the iliohypogastric nerve may be injured.
   b.   For a standard pyelolithotomy, a transverse incision is made in the renal pelvis.
   c.   A successful pyelolithotomy depends on complete mobilization of the kidney.
   d.   The avascular plane of dissection for anatrophic nephrolithotomy generally enters the renal pelvis just anterior to the posterior infundibuli.
   e.   Overdistention of the renal pelvis during coagulum pyelolithotomy may result in pulmonary embolus.

Correct Answer: c   Reference Pages: 704-705
Rationale: For a standard pyelolithotomy, the kidney need not be mobilized any more than necessary to provide exposure to the renal pelvis. A transverse, rather than vertical incision is made to avoid disruption of the functional anatomy of the renal pelvic musculature.

3.   **Which statement regarding complications of stone surgery is incorrect?**

a.   Renal hemorrhage usually occurs within the first 48 hours after surgery.
b.   Pulmonary complications are most common.
c.   Persistent urinary drainage can often be resolved with ureteral stent placement.
d.   Renal deterioration secondary to ischemia is uncommon.
e.   Hypertension rarely occurs.

Correct Answer: a   Reference Pages: 714-715
Rationale: Renal hemorrhage most commonly occurs 7 to 14 days after surgery. It can usually be treated expectantly with fluids and blood transfusions as needed. The antifibrinolytic agent animocaproic acid (Amicar) may also be helpful. Persistent bleeding may require arteriography with selective embolization of the involved vessel or arteriovenous fistula. If bleeding fails to respond to these measures, renal exploration may be required.

4.   **Extensive periureteral dissection during uretolithotomy can cause stricture or even extensive ureteral loss. Which procedure should not be used to manage such complications?**

a.   Boari flap
b.   Psoas hitch
c.   Ileal ureter
d.   Transureteroureterostomy
e.   Ureteral reimplant

Correct Answer: d   Reference Page: 720
Rationale: Transureteroureterostomy should be used in patients with stone disease. If a stone passes down the common ureter, both renal units can be obstructed.

5.   **Which statement concerning instruments for stone fragmentation is incorrect?**

a.   In order to be effective, the top of the ultrasonic probe must be in direct contact with the stone.
b.   Electrohydraulic lithotripsy is more likely to cause ureteral damage than ultrasonic lithotripsy.
c.   Compared to EHL and laser, a disadvantage of ultrasound is that rigid instruments are usually required.
d.   Laser lithotripsy utilizes continuous-wave laser energy.
e.   EHL is useful in fragmenting stones that are resistant to ultrasonic lithotripsy.

Correct Answer: d   Reference Page: 725
Rationale: Laser lithotripsy uses a pulse dye laser that emits laser energy in short bursts with pauses in between. As the laser energy is absorbed by the stone, a plasma

composed of ions and electrons forms at the surface. The plasma is raised to very high pressures and a shock wave results. Tissue damage does not occur unless laser energy is applied for a minimum of 15 seconds. Continuous laser energy cannot be used because excessive temperatures would be required.

6. **Percutaneous nephrolithotomy may be favored over ESWL for all of the following reasons *except*:**

    a.   body habitus of patient.
    b.   renal pelvis stone with associated ureteropelvic junction obstruction.
    c.   cystine calculi.
    d.   stone within a calyceal diverticulum.
    e.   anesthesia risk.

Correct Answer: e   Reference Page: 726

Rationale: Percutaneous nephrolithotomy may be preferred in patients with obesity or kyphoscoliosis because it may be difficult to position the stone in the focal point for ESWL. For patients with an associated UPJ obstruction or a stone in a calyceal diverticulum, passage of gravel from these obstructed systems may not be possible. Patients with an associated ureteropelvic junction obstruction may also undergo simultaneous endopyelotomy at the same time as percutaneous nephrolithotomy. Cystine stones or other stones refractory to ESWL may be better treated with percutaneous techniques. Percutaneous nephrolithotomy requires general anesthesia, whereas newer generation lithotriptors may only require intravenous sedation.

7. **Which statement regarding complications of percutaneous nephrolithotomy is incorrect?**

    a.   The incidence of arteriovenous fistula is less than 1%.
    b.   Management of transcolonic placement of a nephrostomy tube consists of removal of the tube and antibiotics.
    c.   Hemorrhage can usually be controlled with placement of a larger nephrostomy tube.
    d.   Large perforations in the collecting system usually require surgical repair.
    e.   The risk of pneumothorax is low when access is obtained below the 12th rib.

Correct Answer: d   Reference Page: 733

Rationale: Large perforations in the collecting system can usually be managed by nephrostomy tube placement. Complications seldom occur and a nephrostogram in 24 to 36 hours will usually be normal. If a large perforation occurs at the beginning of the procedure, it may be best to terminate the procedure to avoid accumulation of irrigation fluid in the retroperitoneum.

8. **Which statement regarding ureteroscopic stone extraction is true?**

a. A flexible ureteroscope is necessary to reach the proximal ureter.
b. Untreated UTI is an absolute contraindication to ureteroscopy.
c. Ureteral perforation usually requires surgical repair.
d. Ureteral dilation beyond 12F usually results in long-term complications.
e. Ureteroscopy is contraindicated in children.

Correct Answer: b   Reference Page: 736

Rationale: Sterile urine is mandatory before ureteroscopy since irrigation fluid can cause pyelovenous backflow and possible sepsis if the urine is infected.

17
Endourology of the Upper Urinary Tract: Noncalculus Applications

Ralph V. Clayman, Elspeth M. McDougall, R. Sherburne Figenshau

1. **The most common cause of "essential" lateralizing macroscopic hematuria discovered at the time of uretenoscopy is:**

    a. renal cell carcinoma.
    b. transitional cell carcinoma.
    c. renal calculus.
    d. discrete "vascular" lesion.
    e. renal artery aneurysm.

    Correct Answer: d   Reference Page: 752

    Rationale: Patients with essential lateralizing hematuria have by definition already undergone standard imaging tests such as intravenous urography, retrograde ureterography, computed tomography, and/or ultrasonography. These studies can enable the urologist to diagnose the vast majority of cases in which the hematuria is due to a stone or tumor. By the time the patient comes to ureteroscopic evaluation, a discrete bleeding lesion such as a hemangioma or arteriovenous malformation is the most likely underlying problem. Treatment of this lesion leads to long-term cessation of bleeding in over 80% of patients.

2. **Among the following tests for obstruction, which is most associated with a false negative diagnosis of obstruction?**

    a. Diuretic lasix washout renal scan
    b. Intravenous urography
    c. Spiral computed tomography
    d. Whitaker pressure flow test
    e. nephrosonography with resistive indices

    Correct Answer: d   Reference Page: 762

    Rationale: The lasix washout renal scan and the ultrasound study with resistive indices both can result in a false positive diagnosis of UPJ obstruction due to poor renal function or medial renal disease, respectively. Intravenous urography and spiral computed tomography are anatomical and nonfunctional tests; hence, the possibility of a false positive diagnosis of UPJ obstruction is again more likely. However, the Whitaker test, unlike any of the other studies, suffers most from a false negative situation that occurs when there is unnoticed extravasation from the collecting system or when pressure readings are done before the collecting system has been completely filled with contrast.

3. **In which one of the following ureteral strictures would an endoureterotomy have the *highest* chance of being successful?**

a. 2 cm proximal ureteral stricture after failed open pyeloplasty
b. 1 cm middle ureteral stricture following radiation therapy
c. 1 cm left ureteroenteric stricture after cystectomy and ileal conduit diversion for bladder cancer
d. 1 cm stricture in the ureteral tunnel following ureteroscopic stone extraction
e. 2 cm stricture after a radical hysterectomy

Correct Answer: d   Reference Page: 772

Rationale: Endoureterotomy works best on short (< or = 1 cm), nonischemic strictures in the distal or proximal ureter such that one end of the strictured ureter can be marsupialized into the bladder or renal pelvis, respectively. Radiation therapy or radical hysterectomy may lead to ischemic ureteral injury. For ureteroenteric strictures the best success rates are in the 50% to 60% range. Overall, the short, distal nonischemic ureteral stricture fares best; an 80% chance of success can be expected.

4. **A 57-year-old man presents with macroscopic hematuria. An IVP reveals a normal right kidney and a 1 cm filling defect in the renal pelvis of an otherwise normal left kidney. Urine for cytology is negative, and cystoscopy is unremarkable; however, a ureteroscopic biopsy reveals a Grade 2 seemingly noninvasive transitional cell cancer of the renal pelvis. His serum creatinine is 1.2 mg/dl (normal: 0.5 to 1.5 mg/dl). A CT of the abdomen shows only a soft tissue density limited to the left renal pelvis. He is otherwise in excellent health. Your recommended therapy is:**

a. retrograde ureteroscopic resection.
b. percutaneous antegrade resection.
c. 6-week course of retrograde instillation of BCG.
d. nephroureterectomy.
e. open renal exploration, pyelotomy and tumor excision.

Correct Answer: d   Reference Page: 808

Rationale: In a patient with a transitional cell cancer of the renal pelvis and a normal contralateral kidney, nephroureterectomy with a cuff of bladder remains the treatment of choice. Given the multicentricity of renal pelvic TCC and the high local recurrence rates of these tumors, excision of the affected side in patients with a normal contralateral kidney is the most expeditious, and possibly most cost effective therapy.

5.   **In performing an endopyelotomy for a primary UPJ obstruction, the incision should be in which direction?**
a.   Posterior
b.   Anterior
c.   Medial
d.   Lateral
e.   Posteromedial

Correct Answer: d   Reference Page: 787
Rationale: The posterior lateral or straight lateral area of the UPJ is usually the least vascular.

6.   **A 49-year-old man presents with a 2 cm lower pole renal calculus; an IVP reveals that the stone is contained within a 3 cm lower pole calyceal diverticulum. The least morbid, yet highly effective, means for treating the stone and the diverticulum is:**

a.   extracorporeal shock wave lithotripsy (ESWL).
b.   lower pole partial nephrectomy.
c.   retrograde intrarenal ureteroscopic lithotripsy.
d.   upper pole percutaneous nephrostolithotomy.
e.   percutaneous diverticulotomy.

Correct Answer: e   Reference Page: 801
Rationale: Percutaneous direct access into the diverticulum followed by stone removal, incision/dilation of the diverticular neck and fulguration of the walls of the diverticulum offers the best combination of high success and minimal invasion. While lower pole partial nephrectomy is the most efficacious procedure it has a much higher morbidity; in contrast, while ESWL has the lowest morbidity, it also has the poorest success rate, especially given the large size of the stone. Indirect percutaneous access is also associated with a lower success rate; likewise, this would be a difficult area to access ureteroscopically and the stone size would probably preclude achievement of a stone-free state.

7.   **A 64-year-old woman presents with a history of right flank discomfort and new onset hypertension. An ultrasound examination of the kidneys reveals a 4 cm "classic" cyst affecting the lateral border of the lower pole of the right kidney. You recommend:**

a.   laparoscopic cyst decortication.
b.   cyst puncture.
c.   percutaneous drainage and ethanol sclerotherapy.
d.   retrograde intrarenal surgery with ureteroscopic cyst incision.
e.   percutaneous entry into the cyst with endoscopic fulguration of the cyst wall.

Correct Answer: c   Reference Page: 811

Rationale: Percutaneous drainage and ethanol sclerotherapy under intravenous sedation will provide therapeutic cyst ablation in upwards of 97% of patients, at least in the short term. The diagnosis of a "classic" cyst on ultrasound is accurate to the 99% level; if observation were chosen as therapy, there would be no need to proceed with cyst puncture. All of the other forms of "minimally invasive therapy" are more invasive and less successful than percutaneous sclerotherapy.

8. **In which of the following situations after a renal transplant would an endourological approach be most likely to succeed?**

a. Ureteral fistula with ureterovesical disruption
b. Proximal ureteral stricture (1 cm length)
c. Middle ureteral stricture (1 cm length)
d. Distal ureteral stricture (1 cm length)
e. Lymphocele

Correct Answer: d   Reference Page: 814

Rationale: Upwards of 75% of distal ureteral strictures in a renal transplant will respond to endourological therapy, either balloon dilation or endoureterotomy. More proximal ureteral strictures have a response rate of less than 25%. With regard to large ureteral fistulae, an open repair is recommended; however, for the small fistula, an endourologic approach will usually suffice. Lastly, while the majority of post-transplant lymphoceles will respond to drainage (69%), prolonged tube placement may be necessary; 30% will require open or laparoscopic treatment.

18
Laparoscopic Urology
Elspeth McDougall

1. **The use of carbon dioxide as an insufflating gas during laparoscopy may result in which of the following physiologic changes?**

   a. Increased cardiac output
   b. Increased expired end-tidal CO_2
   c. Decreased systemic vascular resistance
   d. Bowel distension
   e. Intraoperative diuresis

   Correct Answer: b   Reference Page: 831
   Rationale: Systemic carbon dioxide absorption during laparoscopy results in a respiratory acidosis and an increase in the expired end-tidal CO_2. Increased abdominal pressure is also associated with a slight decrease in cardiac output and an increase in systemic vascular resistance. Intra-abdominal pressures greater than 10 mmHg have been associated with decreased renal vein flow and oligo-anuria. The only gas that has been used for pneumoperitoneum that may result in bowel distension is nitrous oxide; however, this may occur only in procedures lasting more than an hour.

2. **The increased intra-abdominal pressure associated with a CO_2 pneumoperitoneum may result in all of the following *except*:**

   a. hypercarbia.
   b. systemic acidosis.
   c. elevated ADH levels.
   d. subcutaneous emphysema.
   e. cardiac arrhythmias.

   Correct Answer: c   Reference Pages: 831, 832, 836
   Rationale: Increased intra-abdominal pressure is associated with decrease in renal vein blood flow and concomitant oligoanuria. The increased CO_2 absorption, during insufflation of carbon dioxide into the peritoneal cavity, results in hypercarbia, and a respiratory acidosis. Animal studies have shown that although increased intra-abdominal pressure is associated with decreased renal vein flow and urine output, the quality of the urine, with respect to creatinine clearance and urine osmolality, remain normal; serum ADH levels are not increased.

3. **Veress needle insufflation of the unoperated abdomen is:**

    a.   performed at the umbilicus.
    b.   the safest technique for creating a pneumoperitoneum.
    c.   contraindicated in obese patients.
    d.   quicker than the open, Hasson cannula technique.
    e.   the preferred method of entry in patients with a history of peritonitis.

Correct Answer: a   Reference Page: 832

Rationale: Veress needle insufflation of the abdomen can be performed in any region and has even been described transvaginally through the cul-de-sac. However, the usual site of Veress needle insertion is at the umbilicus which provides the most direct access to the peritoneal cavity because the properitoneal fat and the distance between the skin and the peritoneum are the least. This technique has not been shown to be necessarily quicker than the open Hasson cannula technique. In patients who have had a previous intra-abdominal inflammatory process or multiple surgical procedures, adhesions between the bowel and the anterior abdominal wall may be anticipated and constitute an indication for the open Hasson cannula technique for accessing the abdomen. Overall, in several general surgical series, open access has been found to be safe, yet as quick in creating a pneumoperitoneum as the use of the Veress needle.

4. **During a transperitoneal laparoscopic right nephrectomy in a 280 pound woman, after an hour's work, the right renal vein has been dissected; however, the renal artery still cannot be clearly seen due to overlying and surrounding hilar fat. In addition, the liver edge continues to obscure the field and slow the dissection. Your next step would be:**

    a.   clip and divide the renal vein and proceed to dissect the artery.
    b.   use a variety of retractors to pull the renal vein cephalad or caudal until the renal artery can be seen.
    c.   place an additional 12 mm port to help retract the liver.
    d.   clip and divide the ureter so the hilum can be placed on stretch thereby facilitating dissection of the artery.
    e.   proceed to dissect the posterior surface of the kidney, displace the kidney anteriorly, and dissect the posterior surface of the renal artery.

Correct Answer: e   Reference Pages: 861, 862

Rationale: During a difficult nephrectomy a posterior approach can be most helpful. Approaching the hilum posteriorly allows the surgeon to use gravity to put the renal hilum "on stretch" as the kidney falls medially. Also with this approach, the renal artery presents before the renal vein. Premature occlusion of the vein is ill advised as this may precipitate swelling of the kidney and back-bleeding; the latter may result in the need to convert to an open procedure. Vigorous retraction on the renal vein may likewise result in a venotomy and bleeding. While ureteral and hepatic retraction can be helpful neither will facilitate identification of the renal artery as much as a posterior approach.

5. **The secondary laparoscopic ports are:**

a. placed through the abdominus rectus muscle for trocar stability.
b. not secured to the abdominal wall as laparoscopic visualization eliminates the risk of removing these ports intra-operatively.
c. always a 5 mm port to provide a better cosmetic result for the patient.
d. distributed in a broad arc or circle around the surgical site.
e. always equipped with a safety shield to eliminate the risk of intra-abdominal injury during insertion.

Correct Answer: d   Reference Page: 840

Rationale: All secondary ports are placed under laparoscopic visualization and therefore a safety shield is not absolutely necessary. These ports will facilitate the planned operative procedure by being placed appropriately. Placing the ports lateral to the abdominus rectus muscle will reduce bleeding from the port sites. The size of the port should be determined by the instrumentation that may be required to complete the planned operative procedure; as such 12 mm ports may be needed to accommodate intrapment sacks, vascular staplers, tissue staplers, or hernia clip appliers. All ports should be secured to the abdominal wall so that inadvertent removal during the procedure does not occur.

6. **Termination of the adult laparoscopic procedure includes all of the following *except*:**

a. reduction of the intra-abdominal pressure to 5 mmHg and examination for hemostasis at the operative site and the port sites.
b. removal of all of the ports under direct laparoscopic visualization.
c. closure of the fascia on all ports > 5 mm.
d. release of the CO_2 from the abdomen after removal of the last port.
e. instillation of 500 cc of normal saline with 500 mg of a cephalosporin antibiotic.

Correct Answer: e   Reference Pages: 849, 850

Rationale: It is essential to complete the laparoscopic procedure with an organized plan for exiting the abdomen. This should include desufflation to 5 mmHg pressure to examine for hemostasis, removal of all the ports under laparoscopic visualization, closure of the fascia of all ports greater than 5 mm and release of CO_2 from the abdomen after removal of the last port. Controversy exists as to the use of antibiotics with an irrigating solution; however, clinical studies do not show any advantage to instilling antibiotic solution into the abdomen following the laparoscopic procedure.

Indeed, in the male patient this may result in an uncomfortable, albeit transient, hydrocele.

7.   **The limit of an obturator (limited) pelvic lymph node dissection is in part defined by:**

    a.   the lateral border of the medial umbilical ligament.
    b.   the lateral border of the external iliac vein.
    c.   the genitofemoral nerve.
    d.   Cooper's ligament.
    e.   the spermatic cord.

Correct Answer: a   Reference Page: 850

Rationale: The boundaries of a limited laparoscopic lymph node dissection are: the medial umbilical ligament medially, symphysis pubis caudally, the anterior and medial surfaces of the external iliac vein laterally, the internal iliac vein cranially, and the obturator nerve posteriorly. The genitofemoral nerve defines the lateral border of the extended pelvic lymph node dissection. Neither Cooper's ligament nor the spermatic cord play a role in the dissection boundaries.

8.   **Upon passing the Veress needle at the umbilicus, the CO_2 line is connected. Initial pressure readings are 12 mmHg; after inflow of 200 cc of gas the pressure reading is 15 mmHg. Your next step should be:**

    a.   increase the pressure to 25 mmHg in order to get a larger volume of gas into the abdomen.
    b.   stop the insufflation and push the needle deeper into the abdomen.
    c.   proceed with an open cannula insertion at a different site.
    d.   pass the primary trocar into the peritoneal cavity.
    e.   remove the Veress needle and pass it a second time.

Correct Answer: e   Reference Page: 834

Rationale: During Veress needle insufflation of the abdomen, it is either all right or all wrong. If there is any question as to the appropriate positioning of the Veress needle, it should be removed and reinserted. The five tests confirming intra-peritoneal positioning include: 1) aspiration through the Veress needle with a 10 cc syringe filled with 6 cc of saline should demonstrate gas, 2) injection of a few ccs of the saline should be performed easily, 3) respiration through the Veress needle should yield gas bubbles again, 4) advancement of the Veress needle 1-2 cm into the abdomen should not show any indication of encountering resistance, 5) initial CO_2 insufflation at low flow ($\leq$ 1 L/min) should be associated with an insufflating pressure less than 10 mmHg.

9. **Compared to the open surgical pelvic lymphocelectomy the laparoscopic pelvic lymphocelectomy is:**

   a. of equivalent surgical efficacy.
   b. a quicker procedure to perform.
   c. associated with more postoperative discomfort.
   d. more likely to result in a postoperative ileus.
   e. requires a longer hospital stay and convalescence.

Correct Answer: a   Reference Page: 873

Rationale: Because of decreased patient morbidity and hospitalization, superior cosmesis, and equivalent surgical efficacy, laparoscopic lymphocelectomy is currently viewed as a reasonable alternative to open surgery. Indeed, Gill has noted a lower recurrence rate after laparoscopic therapy. Intraoperative complications such as bladder perforation and injury to the ureter can occur in either technique.

10. **During laparoscopic evaluation of the cryptorchid patient, a blind ending vas deferens is found. The next step is:**

    a. place a second port and explore the area of the psoas muscle and lower pole of the kidney.
    b. terminate the procedure.
    c. proceed to close the inguinal hernia.
    d. make an inguinal incision and look for the testicle along the inguinal canal.
    e. perform a midline incision and proceed with a complete abdominal exploration.

Correct Answer: a   Reference Page: 878, 879

Rationale: Hypoplastic spermatic vessels with a blind ending vas deferens are considered diagnostic of a vanishing testis, implying a congenitally present gonad which underwent torsion or vascular occlusion and resultant ischemic atrophy. Visualization of blind ending spermatic vessels is diagnostic of testicular absence. However, a blind ending vas deferens is not diagnostic of anorchia and mandates a continued search for the testis and spermatic vessels. The presence of an indirect inguinal hernia suggests a viable testis is located within the inguinal canal.

19

Extracorporeal Shock Wave Lithotripsy for the Treatment of Urinary Calculi

Jay Y. Gillenwater

1. **Shock waves can be used to treat urinary calculi because:**

   a. shock waves and ultrasound waves are similar.
   b. shock wave energy is lost during passage to the stone.
   c. focusing shock waves is difficult.
   d. shock waves fragment stones by shear and tear forces.
   e. shock waves' energy is not lost when transmitted through bone.

   Correct Answer: d   Reference Page: 903
   Rationale: Physical properties of shock waves are important basic information to understanding ESWL therapy.

2. **The principal biological effect of ESWL on the kidney is:**

   a. venous rupture.
   b. arterial damage.
   c. calyceal damage.
   d. glomerular damage.
   e. renal tubular damage.

   Correct Answer: a   Reference Page: 905
   Rationale: All the animals show the predominant injury is venous rupture especially of the arcuate veins.

3. **The total number of shocks/per treatment session that is safe during ESWL:**

   a. is related to the incidence of hypertension.
   b. is not defined because safety limits of each machine have not been established.
   c. determines whether you can treat patients with aortic aneurysms.
   d. determines whether you can treat patients with cardiac pacemakers.
   e. is established by the FDA for each machine.

   Correct Answer: b   Reference Page: 905
   Rationale: There have been no studies showing the safe limits of shock waves for each of the machines.

4.   **The most popular method of managing large staghorn calculi is:**

   a.   open surgery.
   b.   ESWL monotherapy.
   c.   percutaneous nephrostolithotomy monotherapy.
   d.   percutaneous nephrostolithotomy plus ESWL.
   e.   surgery plus ESWL.

Correct Answer: d   Reference Page: 909
Rationale: There is no single best therapy but the most popular method is a combination of percutaneous nephrostolithotomy and ESWL because the two procedures are complementary.

5.   **The preferred therapy for a 4 mm mid-ureteral calculus is:**

   a.   push back to the kidney and ESWL.
   b.   ESWL monotherapy.
   c.   ureteroscopy and basket extraction.
   d.   ureteroscopy and lithotripsy with laser or electrohydraulic probe.
   e.   observation for spontaneous passage.

Correct Answer: e   Reference Page: 910
Rationale: Most 4 mm ureteral calculi will pass spontaneously.

6.   **A seven mm ureteral calculi located over the bony pelvis can be treated:**

   a.   by ESWL in the supine position.
   b.   with uretoroscopy and lithotripsy by ultrasound, laser, or electrohydraulic probes.
   c.   by observation because it will usually pass spontaneously.
   d.   by being pushed back to the kidney and treated with ESWL.
   e.   by ureterolithotomy.

Correct Answer: b   Reference Page: 910
Rationale: Bone will block shock waves, 7 mm stones may not pass spontaneously and urethroscopy with lithotripsy would be the preferred therapy by most urologists or ESWL in the prone position.

7.   **When comparing various lithotripters with an artificial stone, the most powerful lithotripter is:**

a.   HM3 - Dornier.
b.   Storz Modulith.
c.   Medstone STS.
d.   EDAP LT01.
e.   MFL-5000 - Dornier.

Correct Answer: b   Reference Page: 915, Fig. 19-3
Rationale: The *in vivo* tests clearly showed the Modulith was the most powerful lithotripter.

20
Renal Cystic Disease
Marguerite C. Lippert

1. **When treating autosomal dominant polycystic kidney disease patients for urinary tract infection, a poor response to antibiotics may suggest all of the following *except*:**

   a. an infected cyst.
   b. an obstructed collecting system.
   c. a lipophobic antibiotic.
   d. hypertension.
   e. the antibiotic has unfavorable activity against infecting organism.

   Correct Answer: d   Reference Page: 928
   Rationale: Urologists are asked to evaluate ADPKD patients with infected cysts and must be familiar with appropriate choices of cyst-penetrating antibiotics and the occasional need to drain an infected cyst.

2. **Similarities between autosomal recessive polycystic kidney disease (ARPKD) and autosomal dominant polycystic kidney disease (ADPKD) in children with symptomatic presentation can include all of the following *except*:**

   a. renomegaly at birth.
   b. hypertension.
   c. renal failure.
   d. no family history of renal cystic disease.
   e. ruptured esophageal varices.

   Correct Answer: e   Reference Page: 923, 930, 931
   Rationale: Since the development of present renal imaging techniques, the number of ADPKD cases discovered in childhood is almost as high as that of ARPKD cases surviving the neonatal period. Hence, distinguishing between the two diseases is not unreasonable. In addition, a negative family history does not eliminate ADPKD.

3. **The following are abdominal CT findings that can be associated with von Hippel-Lindau disease *except*:**

   a. adrenal pheochromocytomas.
   b. hepatic cysts.
   c. pancreatic islet cell tumors, cystadenoma, and cysts.
   d. renal cysts.

e.   renal cell carcinoma.

Correct Answer: b   Reference Page: 936
Rationale: A urologist consulted to evaluate a patient with renal cell carcinoma diagnosed by CT would benefit by knowing other stigmata of von Hippel-Lindau disease so as to potentially diagnose von Hippel-Lindau disease and therefore be able to offer the patient a partial nephrectomy if appropriate.

4.   **Careful study of the contralateral kidney is most important in evaluating a patient with a unilateral multicystic kidney especially to rule out:**

a.   partial duplication.
b.   complete duplication.
c.   vesicoureteral reflux.
d.   nephrolithiasis.
e.   infundibular stenosis.

Correct Answer: c   Reference Page: 940
Rationale: If voiding cystourethrography is routinely performed as a part of the initial evaluation on all infants with a multicystic kidney, up to 28% are found to have contralateral vesicoureteral reflux while only 12% have contralateral UPJ obstruction on ultrasound. Careful study of the contralateral kidney is most important because the prognosis is otherwise excellent.

5.   **CT criteria for a diagnosis of a simple renal cyst include all of the following _except_:**

a.   sharp margination and demarcation from surrounding wall parenchyma.
b.   smooth thin wall.
c.   water density content which is homogeneous throughout.
d.   no enhancement following intravenous contrast administration.
e.   septa.

Correct Answer: e   Reference Page: 945
Rationale: Urologists should be able to evaluate a renal mass by CT and be able to differentiate between simple cyst, complex cyst, and solid mass worrisome for renal cell carcinoma.

6. **The incidence of acquired renal cystic disease in dialysis patients increases with the length of time the patient has received dialysis, but acquired renal cystic disease can be reversed by:**

a. successful renal transplantation.
b. cyclosporin A.
c. erythropoietin.
d. increased kidney weight.
e. decreased kidney weight.

Correct Answer: a   Reference Page: 951

Rationale: Urologists should understand that acquired renal cystic disease (ARCD) has a rising incidence with increasing duration of uremia or dialysis but that the cysts of ARCD can be reversible with successful renal transplantation.

21
Hydronephrosis
Jay Y. Gillenwater

1.   The part of the kidney the least damaged by hydronephrosis is:

    a. distal tubule.
    b. proximal tubule.
    c. loop of Henle.
    d. glomeruli.
    e. collecting tubule.

Correct Answer: d   Reference Page: 963
Rationale: Glomerular changes are the last ones to occur during hydronephrosis.

2.   Renal compensatory hypertrophy occurs after unilateral ureteral obstruction:

    a. to bring total renal function back to normal.
    b. within a few minutes.
    c. because of an unknown renotrophic factor.
    d. because of obligatory growth factors.
    e. causing only hypertrophy and no hyperplasia.

Correct Answer: c   Reference Page: 964
Rationale: Renal compensatory hypertrophy is caused by an unknown humoral stimulus and does not bring function back to normal.

3.   The human kidney cannot regain function after complete obstruction for:

    a. 3 days.
    b. 7 days.
    c. 21 days.
    d. 80 days.
    e. 180 days.

Correct Answer: d   Reference Page: 965
Rationale: The longest reported return of function after complete obstruction is 69 days.

4.   The principal physiological alteration during chronic hydronephrosis is:

    a. high renal pelvic pressures.
    b. low renal blood flow because of preglomerular vasoconstriction.

c.   venous vasoconstriction.
d.   postglomerular vasoconstriction causing low renal blood flow.
e.   tubular-glomeruli backflow.

Correct Answer: b   Reference Page: 967
Rationale: The principal long-term physiologic change is preglomerular vasoconstriction by some unexplained physiological mechanism.

5.   **Short-term ureteral obstruction most severely damages:**

a.   sodium reabsorption.
b.   chloride reabsorption.
c.   urinary dilution.
d.   urinary concentrating ability.
e.   potassium excretion.

Correct Answer: d   Reference Page: 969
Rationale: Urinary concentrating ability is the first and earliest renal function damaged by obstruction.

6.   **Clinical postobstructive diuresis is:**

a.   seen frequently with release of unilateral ureteral obstruction.
b.   is a common clinical problem in BPH.
c.   is physiologic, usually mild and self-limiting.
d.   caused by over-response to ADH.
e.   caused by over-response to aldosterone.

Correct Answer: c   Reference Page: 971
Rationale: Most postobstructive diuresis is mild and fluid replacement is controlled by the thirst mechanism if the patient is conscious.

7.   **The best method to determine if a dilated upper tract is obstructed is:**

a.   intravenous urogram.
b.   ultrasound.
c.   renal scan.
d.   CT scan.
e.   MRI.

Correct Answer: c   Reference Page: 972
Rationale: A physiological test is necessary to verify that a dilated upper tract is obstructed, not an anatomic study.

22
Renal Transplant

Ernest E. Hodge, Stuart M. Flechner, Andrew C. Novick

1. **Which of the following conditions in a potential recipient represent an absolute contraindication to renal transplantation?**

    a. Coronary artery disease
    b. Active infection
    c. History of malignancy
    d. Diverticulosis
    e. Benign prostatic hypertrophy

    Correct Answer: b   Reference Pages: 1019, 1020
    Rationale: While the other conditions may represent relative contraindications and require intervention and correction prior to transplantation, they do not represent an absolute contraindication. Also, a history of malignancy may require a mandatory waiting period following treatment prior to transplantation.

2. **The "routine" urologic evaluation of a potential transplant recipient will include all of the following *except*:**

    a. thorough history.
    b. complete physical examination.
    c. urinalysis and urine culture.
    d. voiding cystourethrogram.
    e. cystoscopy.

    Correct Answer: e   Reference Pages: 1017, 1018
    Rationale: The routine urologic evaluation of potential transplant recipients will usually not include a cystoscopy. The evaluation may include additional urologic procedures including cystoscopy, bilateral retrograde pyelograms, urodynamic studies, etc. if specific indications are identified in the history, physical examination, examination of the urine or on the voiding cystourethrogram. In fact, some centers are now questioning the need for routine VCUG in patients with good urine output and no urologic symptoms.

3. **Presence in the donor of which of the following will most likely result in permanent renal injury with a poor outcome following transplantation?**

    a. Prolonged cold ischemia (greater than 24 hours)
    b. Anuria with a rising serum creatinine

c. Prolonged hypotension (BP < or = to 90 mm HG)
d. Warm ischemia
e. Administration of nephrotoxic antibiotics

Correct Answer: a   Reference Page: 1026

Rationale: Although the factors described above can aggravate acute tubular necrosis in the donor kidney, the combination of a rising creatinine and a markedly diminished urine output is associated with permanent renal injury and would signify the highest risk of poor outcome following transplantation. Thus, the goal of donor maintenance would be to hopefully reverse any ATN establishing a stable or decreasing serum creatinine and adequate urine output at the time of donor nephrectomy.

4. **Which of the following immunosuppressive agents is least effective in the treatment of acute cellular rejection?**

   a. High dose oral steroids
   b. Polyclonal antilymphocyte agents (MALG, etc.)
   c. Monoclonal antilymphocyte agents (OKT3, etc.)
   d. Cyclosporine
   e. Intravenous steroids

Correct Answer: d   Reference Pages: 1011, 1042, 1043

Rationale: While early initial reports suggested that cyclosporine may be of benefit in the treatment of acute cellular rejection, it has not proven to be an effective agent for the treatment of an existing rejection episode. Cyclosporine's role has been established as that of an induction/maintenance agent in the prevention of rejection.

5. **The most common etiology of ureteral fistula following renal transplantation is:**

   a. surgical technical error.
   b. ureteral ischemia with necrosis.
   c. rejection.
   d. bladder outlet obstruction.
   e. urinary tract infection.

Correct Answer: b   Reference Pages: 1051-1053

Rationale: A compromise of the ureteral vascularity with subsequent necrosis and sloughing is the most common cause of post transplant ureteral fistula. A few fistulas, in the immediate post-operative period, are the result of technical error, while a rare fistula may be the result of obstruction or infection.

6.   A 32-year-old male is three months post-renal transplant. He presents with the acute onset of 2+ ipsilateral scrotal and lower extremity edema, an increase in the size of the kidney by palpation and an elevation of his serum creatinine from 1.6 to 2.4 mg/%. Which of the following would be the most appropriate initial diagnostic study?

a.   Cystogram
b.   Renal transplant ultrasound
c.   Intravenous pyelogram
d.   Renal transplant biopsy
e.   Renal transplant angiogram.

Correct Answer: b   Reference Page: 1054
Rationale: The physical findings described in this scenario are most consistent with a post-transplant lymphocele and a renal transplant ultrasound demonstrating a perinephric fluid collection with hydronephrosis would be the most revealing initial diagnostic study. Subsequently, a diagnostic aspiration of the fluid or CT scan with contrast to exclude a urine fistula may be appropriate.

7.   Currently, the most common cause of hypertension following renal transplantation is:

a.   native kidney renin production.
b.   vasomotor effects of cyclosporine.
c.   chronic rejection.
d.   transplant renal artery stenosis.
e.   recurrent glomerulonephritis in the transplanted kidney.

Correct Answer: b   Reference Page: 1046
Rationale: Prior to the routine use of cyclosporine, renin mediated causes related to the native kidney and chronic rejection were the most common causes of post transplant hypertension. However, direct effects of cyclosporine are now the single most common contributing factor to hypertension following transplantation.

23

Renovascular Hypertension

R. Ernest Sosa and E. Darracott Vaughan, Jr.

1. **Renin is secreted in response to which stimuli?**

    a. Increased mean arterial pressure, increased sodium intake and low plasma aldosterone levels
    b. Decreased salt intake and a drop in blood pressure
    c. High plasma aldosterone levels
    d. Beta blockers
    e. Change in position from upright to supine

    Correct Answer: b   Reference Page: 1061

    Rationale: The principal stimulants of renin secretion are a decreased sodium (or chloride) load reaching the macula densa, low renal perfusion pressure at the baroreceptors in the afferent arteriole and beta-1 stimulation of the juxtaglomerular cells.

2. **A 60-year-old white male is found to have a blood pressure of 190/100 mm Hg. His last blood pressure determination one year ago revealed a blood pressure of 150/90. He is asymptomatic. On physical examination he has no fundic exudates, hemorrhages or papilledema. Bruits are heard over his left carotid artery and in the mid-epigastric area. His BUN and serum creatinine are normal. His urinalysis is free of protein and cells. Repeat examination reveals the hypertension is sustained. The next step in his evaluation would include:**

    a. a trial on diuretics to control his blood pressure.
    b. duplex ultrasonography to evaluate his bruits.
    c. a rapid sequence excretory pyelogram.
    d. an ambulatory peripheral renin indexed to a 24-hour urine sodium.
    e. a stress test to see if he has coronary artery disease.

    Correct Answer: d   Reference Page: 1065

    Rationale: This patient has undergone a significant and sustained increase in blood pressure over the past year. He has bruits in the mid-epigastrium and over the carotid artery suggesting diffuse atherosclerotic disease. Renovascular hypertension is strongly suggested and must be ruled out. A trial of diuretics will only serve to increase renin secretion from the ischemic kidney secondary to sodium depletion and will not control the hypertension. The duplex ultrasound may reveal a renal artery narrowing with decreased flow but will not establish a causal relation between the renovascular disease and the hypertension. An excretory urogram is likely to have a high rate of false positive and false negative findings. An elevated peripheral plasma renin indexed against a 24-hour urine sodium is a reliable screening test for renovascular hypertension.

3. **The peripheral plasma renin in the above patient is 5.2, indexed to a 24-hour urine sodium of 84. On the single dose captopril test his peripheral renin increased to 20 ng/ml/hr. Angiography reveals a normal right renal artery and an 80% stenosis of the left renal artery, not involving the ostium. His electrocardiogram and stress test are normal and he has minimal carotid artery disease. The next step in this patient's management should be:**

   a. renal vein renin sampling with and without captopril.
   b. a trial of converting enzyme inhibitors.
   c. weight reduction and low salt diet.
   d. splenorenal bypass.
   e. percutaneous renal artery angioplasty.

   Correct Answer: a   Reference Page: 1072
   Rationale: Renal vein renins can be measured in the outpatient setting to confirm the presence of renin-dependent hypertension and to predict curability before beginning treatment.

4. **Renal vein renin samples measured in a patient with renal artery stenosis off all medications for three weeks are as follows:**

left renal vein	**10 ng/ml/hr**
inferior vena cava	**8 ng/ml/hr**
right renal vein	**8 ng/ml/hr**
inferior vena cava	**8 ng/ml/hr**

   These studies indicate that:

   a. the patient doesn't have renovascular hypertension.
   b. a captopril challenge would not affect these values.
   c. this is an inadequate study and should be repeated.
   d. this patient has essential hypertension and should be treated with diuretics.
   e. the patient did not stop all of his medicines.

   Correct Answer: c   Reference Page: 1071
   Rationale: Sealey (1973) showed that in order to maintain a steady level of renin activity, a 25% increment in renin must be contributed by each kidney when renal arteriovenous differences are compared. The renal vein renin measurements in this example do not fulfill this criterion, and suggest a sampling error was committed, requiring repeat sampling.

5.   **In comparison to atherosclerotic renal artery occlusions, fibromuscular diseases of the renal artery:**

a.   do not progress.
b.   do not have lasting benefit from angioplasty.
c.   do not dissect or thrombose.
d.   are more likely to involve other major arteries.
e.   usually occur in a younger age group.

Correct Answer: e   Reference Page: 1060

Rationale: Fibromuscular diseases occur in a younger age group than atherosclerotic disease but can be associated with progressive stenosis, dissection, and obstruction of one or both renal arteries. Fibromuscular diseases respond well to balloon dilation.

6.   **Surgical renal revascularization is contraindicated:**

a.   in diffuse aortic atherosclerosis.
b.   in the presence of coexistent coronary artery disease.
c.   if the blood pressure is well controlled by medication.
d.   in elderly patients.
e.   in azotemic patients.

Correct Answer: b   Reference Page: 1079

Rationale: Renal revascularization in patients with significant coronary artery disease is associated with increased morbidity and mortality. Diffuse aortic atherosclerosis is not a contraindication to revascularization. Hepatorenal and splenorenal bypass surgery are good alternatives to aortorenal bypass in this setting. Azotemia can often be stabilized or improved by renal revascularization. Despite adequate blood pressure control with medical management, continued decrease in renal function and renal loss occur.

24
The Ureter
Robert M. Weiss, Bo L.R.A. Coolsaet

1. **The electrical activity of the ureter and other smooth muscles depends on the distribution of ions across the cell membrane and on the relative permeability of the cell membrane to these ions. During the resting state the:**

    a. concentration of K^+ ions is higher on the outside of the cell membrane.
    b. concentration of Na^+ ions is higher on the inside of the cell membrane.
    c. cell membrane is preferentially permeable to K^+.
    d. cell membrane is preferentially permeable to Na^+.
    e. inside of the cell membrane is positive with respect to the outside of the cell membrane.

    Correct Answer: c   Reference Page: 1102
    Rationale: During the resting state the cell membrane is preferentially permeable to K^+ and the tendency of K^+ to move from the inside of the cell where it is more concentrated to the outside of the cell membrane creates an electrical gradient across the cell membrane with the inside of the cell membrane being negative with respect to the outside.

2. **Of the following agents, the one most likely to inhibit ureteral activity is:**

    a. phenylephrine.
    b. nifedipine.
    c. acetylcholine.
    d. substance P.
    e. propranolol.

    Correct Answer: b   Reference Page: 1116
    Rationale: Phenylephrine is an alpha-adrenergic agonist, acetylcholine is a muscarinic cholinergic agonist and substance P is a tachykinin and all stimulate ureteral smooth muscle. Propranolol is a beta-adrenergic antagonist and blocks the inhibitory effects of beta-adrenergic agonists such as isoproterenol. Nifedipine is a calcium channel blocker and inhibits the inward movement of calcium across the cell membrane which is needed for the upstroke of the ureteral action potential and for supplying the calcium that is required for the contractility.

3.   **The Laplace relationship provides a rationale for ureteral tapering, but more importantly, a rationale for the use of augmentation cystoplasties and low pressure urinary reservoirs. The Laplace relationship states that:**

   a.   pressure = stress/force.
   b.   pressure = (radius x wall thickness)/stress.
   c.   pressure = force/stress.
   d.   pressure = force/(radius x wall thickness).
   e.   pressure = (stress x wall thickness)/radius.

Correct Answer: e   Reference Page: 1107
Rationale: Stress equals force/unit area and thus A and C are incorrect. Pressure decreases when a force is distributed over a large area; thus B is incorrect. A thicker wall structure should increase pressure; thus the correct answer is e.

4.   **Nitric oxide is involved in smooth muscle relaxation. The second messenger involved in that action is:**

   a.   inositol triphosphate (IP$_3$).
   b.   cyclic AMP.
   c.   diacylglycerol.
   d.   cyclic GMP.
   e.   L-arginine.

Correct Answer: d   Reference Page: 1115
Rationale: Nitric oxide activates the enzyme guanylyl cyclase with the formation of cyclic GMP that results in smooth muscle relaxation. L-arginine is the substrate for nitric oxide formation.

5.   **Two factors that are most beneficial for ureteral stone passage are:**

   a.   increased intraluminal hydrostatic pressure and ureteral relaxation.
   b.   decreased intraluminal hydrostatic pressure and ureteral relaxation.
   c.   increased ureteral peristaltic frequency and increased intraluminal hydrostatic pressure.
   d.   decreased ureteral peristaltic frequency and increased intraluminal hydrostatic pressure.
   e.   decreased intraluminal hydrostatic pressure and increased ureteral contractile force.

Correct Answer: a   Reference Page: 1110
Rationale: Ureteral relaxation in the region of the calculus is the most important factor in stone passage. The hydrostatic pressure load also aids in stone passage.

6. **Theophylline is a smooth muscle relaxant. Theophylline:**

   a.   activates adenylyl cyclase.
   b.   activates guanylyl cyclase.
   c.   inhibits phosphodiesterase.
   d.   inhibits protein kinase C.
   e.   blocks IP_3 production.

Correct Answer: c   Reference Page: 1114
Rationale: Theophylline inhibits the enzyme phosphodiesterase which degrades the second messenger cyclic AMP. This results in an increase in cyclic AMP and smooth muscle relaxation.

7. **Calmodulin:**

   a.   activates myosin.
   b.   activates myosin light chain kinase.
   c.   is more active in its phosphorylated form.
   d.   is a second messenger.
   e.   is a calcium binding protein.

Correct Answer: e   Reference Page: 1104
Rationale: Calmodulin is a protein that is present in many cell types. Without calcium, calmodulin is inactive. Upon binding with calcium it forms an active complex that can activate enzymes involved in the contractile process.

25
Diseases of the Retroperitoneum
M. Craig Hall

1. **Which of the following statements concerning primary retroperitoneal sarcomas is true?**

   a. A well defined pseudocapsule facilitates complete resection.
   b. Following complete resection, local recurrence is unusual.
   c. Tumor grade and completeness of resection are the most significant predictors of survival.
   d. Patients typically become symptomatic before these tumors reach considerable size.
   e. Despite complete resection, most patients ultimately succumb to distant metastatic disease.

   Correct Answer: c   Reference Page: 1135
   Rationale: Primary retroperitoneal sarcomas tend to be locally aggressive neoplasms that reach considerable size prior to diagnosis. Tumor grade and the completeness of tumor resection are the most reliable predictors of ultimate survival. Sarcomas invariably extend beyond their pseudocapsule, and dissection should be carried out well beyond its limits. Despite microscopic and even pathologic complete resection, local recurrence rates of 35% to 79% at 5 years are reported. Only approximately one-third of patients will ever develop distant metastatic disease with progressive local regional disease occurring in 75% of patients.

2. **Primary retroperitoneal sarcomas tend to be locally aggressive neoplasms:**

   a. that metastasize principally by lymphatic spread.
   b. that often require the en bloc resection of adjacent organs for complete resection.
   c. for which effective chemotherapy has significantly improved outcome.
   d. that are associated with viral transformation in humans.
   e. that also have a propensity for early hematogenous dissemination.

   Correct Answer: b   Reference Page: 1129
   Rationale: Though primary retroperitoneal sarcomas tend to be locally aggressive, lymphatic metastases are uncommon at the time of initial diagnosis. These tumors metastasize principally by the hematogenous route. Although several clinical conditions are associated with the development of sarcomas, there is no known association with viral transformation in humans. The removal of adjacent organs is

often required to obtain a complete resection. Though commonly employed, systemic chemotherapy has not clearly been shown to improve outcome.

3.   **A 55-year-old woman with bilateral hydronephrosis and a creatinine of 2.8 as a result of retroperitoneal fibrosis has bilateral ureteral stents placed at the time of retrograde pyelography. Following a short trial of corticosteroids, CT scan demonstrates near-resolution of the fibrous plaque and ureteral encasement. The next step in management is:**

a.   supravesical urinary diversion.
b.   exploratory laparotomy with multiple deep biopsies to rule out malignant disease and bilateral ureteral lysis.
c.   discontinuing the corticosteroids and repeating the CT scan in 4 weeks.
d.   thin needle biopsy in the area of the previous fibrous plaque.
e.   removal of the ureteral stents and close follow-up with monitoring of renal function and the status of the upper urinary tracts.

Correct Answer: e   Reference Pages: 1142-1143
Rationale: Following the establishment of urinary tract drainage, corticosteroid therapy may be effective as initial primary treatment for patients with retroperitoneal fibrosis. One must always maintain a high index of suspicion for a malignant etiology and rule out malignant disease when suggested and when there is little response to a short trial of corticosteroids. Retroperitoneal fibrosis has a propensity for relapse and therefore close long-term follow-up is mandatory.

4.   **Pelvic lipomatosis is a poorly understood clinicopathologic entity that is characterized by an abnormal proliferation of fibroadipose tissue in the pelvis. Characteristically:**

a.   there is no racial predominance.
b.   two-thirds of patients are female.
c.   patients present most commonly with gastrointestinal complaints; urologic symptoms are unusual.
d.   most patients can be managed conservatively with intervention reserved for complications, primarily obstructive uropathy.
e.   a large percentage of patients have cystitis glandularis that progresses to adenocarcinoma in up to 25% of patients.

Correct Answer: d   Reference Page: 1145 and 1148
Rationale: Over 90% of patients reported with lipomatosis have been men, and two-thirds have been black. Although GI complaints are frequent, up to three-fourths of patients also have urinary symptoms and signs at presentation. Most patients can be managed conservatively; however, a significant proportion will require operative intervention for the management of complications, most com-

monly, ureteral obstruction. A large percentage of patients with pelvic lipomatosis are found to have cystitis glandularis. These patients may be at an increased risk for the development of adenocarcinoma, but this is a rare occurrence.

5.   **Which of the following statements concerning retroperitoneal fibrosis is true?**

    a.   Most cases can be attributed to a specific etiology.
    b.   The disease is 2-3 times more common in women than in men.
    c.   Retrograde stenting of the ureters is usually not possible.
    d.   Cessation of the offending drug usually results in prompt resolution of the inflammatory process.
    e.   Multiple deep biopsies of the fibrous plaque at the time of ureterolysis are important to rule out malignant disease.

Correct Answer: e   Reference Pages: 1137, 1140, 1143
Rationale: Approximately two-thirds of cases of retroperitoneal fibrosis are idiopathic, and the disease is 2 to 3 times more common in men. Characteristically, despite narrowing and deviation of the ureters, one can usually pass a stent retrograde beyond the area of obstruction. Although stopping the offending drug has been reported to result in resolution of the process, this is probably uncommon, and progression may even be seen. One should always have a high index of suspicion for ruling out malignant disease and perform biopsies as necessary in order to rule it out.

6.   **A 46-year-old man on Coumadin for a previous deep venous thrombosis has right flank and abdominal pain. There is no history of trauma. Subsequent CT scan is normal except for a large right perirenal hematoma. His hemoglobin remains stable at 9.7 over the next 48 hours. Arteriography is normal. The next step in management is:**

    a.   exploratory laparotomy with evacuation of the hematoma and right nephrectomy.
    b.   flank exploration, evacuation of hematoma, and nephrectomy.
    c.   flank exploration, evacuation of hematoma, and drainage of the perirenal space.
    d.   cystoscopy and retrograde pyelogram.
    e.   Follow-up serial CT scans with pre- and post-contrast thin cuts through the adrenal and renal beds.

Correct Answer: e   Reference Page: 1152-1153

Rationale: Spontaneous retroperitoneal hemorrhage in the absence of trauma or a ruptured abdominal aortic aneurysm is often related to pathology involving the adrenal gland or kidney. In fact, the majority of cases are associated with benign and malignant tumors of the kidney. With modern imaging techniques, including CT scan and arteriography, the underlying cause can be determined before surgical exploration in most cases. Pre- and post-contrast CT scans should be obtained with thin cuts taken through the adrenal and renal beds. When a mass is not clearly detected, follow-up scans may allow the detection of small renal neoplasms which may have been previously obscured by the presence of the hematoma. In the case discussed above, this represents the most appropriate next step in management and may thereby avoid unnecessary exploration with a high attendant risk of removal of a potentially normal kidney.

26A
Voiding Function: Relevant Anatomy, Physiology, Pharmacology, and Molecular Aspects

Stephen A. Zderic, Robert M. Levin, Alan J. Wein

1. **Which of the following statements best describes the basis for the bladder's remarkable compliance?**

    a. Bladder compliance is a function of the extracellular matrix.

    b. Bladder compliance is determined by cytosolic calcium levels within the cytosol of the smooth muscle.

    c. Bladder compliance is the sum of interactions between the intracellular components of the smooth muscle cells, extracellular matrix, and the autonomic nervous system.

    d. Bladder compliance is dramatically influenced by the actions of the autonomic nervous system.

    e. Bladder compliance is determined by the combination of cytoskeletal fibers and an anatomic realignment of the smooth muscle cells during filling.

Correct Answer: c   Reference Page: See rationale.

Rationale: Each of these statements contains a true fact(s); however it is answer C which best summarizes what is known today about bladder compliance. The bladder is the most compliant organ within the body in terms of its ability to undergo remarkable expansion at a low storage pressure, and then empty over 95% of its volume. The bladder's ability to store urine at low pressures is related to the extracellular matrix, although this relationship is complex and still not well understood (pages 1206-1207). The bladder smooth muscle cells require appropriate amounts of cytosolic calcium to maintain proper tone as shown by the experiments of Coplen et al (Fig 26A-14). The autonomic nervous system also contributes to bladder tone, and is in turn modulated by supraspinal influences (page 1202). The cytoskeletal filaments including actin and myosin are important in maintaining cell shape which will be distorted during filling and the cells change their shape (pages 1165-1166). Furthermore the polymerization of such fibers is calcium sensitive. However it is statement (c) which provides the best answer because it acknowledges the importance of the 3 major contributors to compliance.

2.   **Which of the following statements best describes the distribution of cholinergic and adrenergic receptors within the bladder?**

   a.   The highest alpha receptor density is in the bladder body (dome).
   b.   The body (dome) is rich in cholinergic and contains some beta adrenergic receptors.
   c.   The body (dome) is rich in beta adrenergic receptors and contains some cholinergic receptors.
   d.   The body (dome) contains cholinergic receptors.
   e.   The bladder base is rich in beta adrenergic receptors.

Correct Answer: b   Reference Page: 1188, 1191

Rationale: The distribution of autonomic receptors within the bladder is best summarized as follows (pages 1188 & 1191). The bladder body is richly innervated with cholinergic innervation, and here the muscle expresses the highest concentration of cholinergic receptors. The clinical relevance of this fact is that this is the site where anticholinergic medications exert their effects. Within the body, there are also found beta adrenergic receptors. These are involved in supressing muscle contractility and in vitro are capable of smooth muscle relaxation. Clinically these beta receptors do not respond to beta blockers in a way that induces a measurable urodynamic effect. The highest alpha receptor density is found in the bladder base, and it is these receptors which mediate the constriction of the trigonal fibers. Statements a,c, and e are false. Statement d is correct, but it is answer b that is most accurate.

3.   **Which of the following statements about the neurochemistry of cotransmitters is most accurate?**

   a.   The clinical relevance of cotransmitters such as ATP is that even in the presence of an anticholinergic drug such as oxybutynin, uninhibited contractions (although of lesser intensity) may occur.
   b.   Nitric oxide has been shown to have no effect on the bladder outlet and a major effect on the bladder body.
   c.   The only function of ATP is to serve as a source of intracellular energy which maintains ionic gradients within the neuron.
   d.   One neuron secretes one neurotransmitter.
   e.   A cotransmitter is an agent secreted by one neuron which modulates the action of an adjacent neuron.

Correct Answer: a   Reference Page: 1189

Rationale: The concept of a coneurotransmitter is one with clinical relevance to a urologist using pharmacologic therapy to enhance bladder capacity and improve continence. One neuron may secrete more than one neurotransmitter, and release these products into the synaptic cleft. For example, ATP and nitric oxide have both been shown to be released by neurons which also have the capacity to secrete acetylcholine (page 1189). Statement b is false: nitric oxide does play a role in the relaxation of bladder base smooth muscle in experimental systems, with a minimal role in the bladder body. Statement c is also false in that ATP was described by Burnstock in 1972 as a neurotransmitter which is secreted out of the neuron and into the synapse. It is true that ATP is the source of energy for the Na^+-K^+ ATPase which sites on the neuron's surface and maintains the electrical potential. Statements d and e are false as discussed above.

4. **Which of the following statements about the pontine micturition center and central nervous system control of bladder function is most accurate?**

    a. Gamma-aminobutyric acid (GABA) is an excitatory neurotransmitter within the spinal cord and the pontine micturition center.

    b. The pontine micturition center serves to contract the bladder outlet and thereby facilitates urinary storage.

    c. Uninhibited bladder contractions are diminished if the lumbosacral cord is removed or ganglionic neurotransmission is blocked with hexamethonium.

    d. Interruptions in the cortical tracts leading to the pontine micturition center produce contraction of the external striated sphincter with simultaneous contraction of the detrusor (detrusor sphincter dyssynergia).

    e. Through the neurotransmitters gamma-aminobutyric acid (GABA) and glutamate, the pontine micturition center exerts a tonic inhibitory influence over the parasympathetic nuclei within the sacral cord segments (Onuf's nucleus).

Correct Answer: e   Reference Page: 1202-1203

Rationale: The pontine micturition center consists of a nucleus within the brain stem that serves to produce a chronic inhibitory influence over the sacral parasympathetic nuclei (which serve to initiate a bladder contraction). The neurons within the spinal cord that convey this inhibitory signal utilize GABA and glutamate as their primary transmitters. With activation of the pontine micturition center by cortical input, this inhibitory effect is lost, and the sacral parasympathetic nuclei (Onuf's nucleus) are stimulated to initiate the cholinergic transmission that results in a bladder contraction (pages 1202-1203). Answer a is incorrect in that GABA serves as an inhibitory transmitter. Answer b is wrong in that the pontine center does not directly affect the smooth muscle at the bladder outlet. Answer c is wrong because the presence of uninhibited bladder contractions in experimental animal models is increased by removal of the lumbosacral cord or the application of hexamethonium (a ganglionic blocking agent). Answer d is wrong because interruptions of the cortical tracts produce uninhibited contractions of the bladder, but the process of micturition does occur with synergy.

26B
Voiding Dysfunction: Diagnosis, Classification, and Management
William D. Steers

1. **Possesses anticholinergic activity, direct smooth muscle inhibitory activity, and local anesthetic properties:**

   a. baclofen.
   b. oxbutynin.
   c. propantheline.
   d. hyoscyamine.
   e. DMSO.

   Correct Answer: b   Reference Page: 1318
   Rationale: Oxbutynin possess anticholinergic, direct smooth muscle inhibitory activity and local anesthetic properties. Its ability to decrease bladder contractility is the result of these actions. Baclofen and propantheline are anticholinergic agents. Baclofen has significantly greater ganglionic blocking action than does propantheline. Hyoscyamine is an anticholinergic/antispasmodic drug and is one of the components of belladonna alkaloids. Terodiline is a calcium channel blocker with antimuscarinic properties.

2. **An interrupted flow pattern on a voiding flow rate study suggests:**

   a. urethral stricture.
   b. detrusor hyperreflexia.
   c. detrusor sphincter dyssynergia.
   d. internal sphincter dyssynergia.
   e. autonomic dysreflexia.

   Correct Answer: c   Reference Page: 1289
   Rationale: The voiding flow rate is often a useful screening measure especially in children to indicate whether problems exist with a bladder outlet. Internal sphincter dyssynergia, because of smooth muscle, would not have a time course enough to interrupt the stream and would most likely appear as an obstructed low flow pattern similar to that of BPH.

3.   **An external sphincter EMG is used to assess:**

    a.   potentials generated by striated external sphincter muscle.
    b.   whether pudendal afferents are intact.
    c.   outlet resistance in midurethral pressure zone.
    d.   pudendal nerve function.
    e.   coordination of the bladder with its outlet.

Correct Answer: a   Reference Page: 1290

Rationale: EMG activity measures potentials. b) is incorrect since afferents can be destroyed and EMG still has activity; c) pressure cannot be measured so outlet resistance cannot be ascertained; d) with denervation the external sphincter EMG may still show denervation potentials, which are not directly correlated whether the pudendal nerve is intact; e) coordination of bladder with its outlet can only be obtained by a combination of CMG and EMG.

4.   **Combined pressure/uroflow study is used to diagnose:**

    a.   prostatism.
    b.   function of bladder outlet.
    c.   function of bladder and its outlet.
    d.   site of obstruction.
    e.   impaired contractility.

Correct Answer: c   Reference Page: 1297

Rationale: Pressure flow study is the gold standard to determine if obstruction exists. It represents a combined effect of both the bladder and its outlet. It does not identify the site of obstruction. Prostatism is a symptom complex not always related to degree of obstruction. A pressure flow study in many instances cannot determine if low detrusor pressure is due to impaired contractility or obstruction.

5.   **A pure lower motoneuron lesion to the bladder is associated with:**

    a.   spastic lower limbs.
    b.   detrusor areflexia.
    c.   a hyperreflexic bladder.
    d.   non-relaxation of the external striated urethral sphincter.
    e.   a positive bulbocavernosus reflex.

Correct Answer: b   Reference Page: 1343

Rationale: The lower motoneuron lesion is suggested by a neurologic examination showing an absent bulbocavernosus reflex. Flaccid striated muscles and paralysis below the level of the lesion are seen. Detrusor areflexia is also seen. Spastic lower limbs, hyperreflexic bladder, a non-relaxing external sphincter, and positive bulbocavernosus reflex are indicative of an upper motoneuron lesion.

6.   **To distinguish true sphincter dyssynergia from pseudodyssynergia due to voluntary contraction of the external sphincter, the most useful measurement is:**

   a.   intravesical pressure.
   b.   striated sphincter EMG.
   c.   maximum urethral pressure.
   d.   rectal pressure.
   e.   urine flow rate.

Correct Answer: d   Reference Page: 1296

Rationale: It is difficult or impossible by combining CMB and EMG to distinguish voluntary contraction of the external sphincter from true sphincter dyssynergia. The most helpful measure listed would be indirect measurement of the intra-abdominal pressure by recording rectal pressure. This would tell whether a patient is voluntarily straining. Investigators have suggested that the time of onset of the EMG signal relative to the rate of rise of bladder pressure would be useful to distinguish voluntary from involuntary contraction of the external urethral sphincter.

7.   **Augmentation cystoplasty is most useful in the treatment of:**

   a.   radiation cystitis.
   b.   interstitial cystitis.
   c.   intrinsic sphincter deficiency.
   d.   reduced bladder compliance.
   e.   detrusor areflexia.

Correct Answer: d   Reference Page: 1325

Rationale: Augmentation cystoplasty would be contraindicated with radiation cystitis because of poor wound healing and susceptibility to spontaneous rupture. While augmentation cystoplasty has been used to treat interstitial cystitis, multiple studies report poor efficacy. It has been shown that in myelodysplastic children, augmentation cystoplasty fails to correct underlying intrinsic sphincter deficiency and urinary incontinence remains. Detrusor areflexia may be associated with poor bladder compliance, but in itself is not an indication for augmentation cystoplasty. The only reasonable answer is reduced bladder compliance. Reducing leak point pressure below 40 cm of water preserves upper tracts and represents the single best indication for this procedure.

8. **Combined urethral hypermobility (type II stress urinary incontinence) and intrinsic sphincter deficiency (type III stress urinary incontinence) are best treated by:**

    a.   suprapubic bladder suspension.
    b.   vaginal bladder suspension.
    c.   alpha-adrenergic agonists.
    d.   intravaginal estrogens.
    e.   pubovaginal fascial sling.

Correct Answer: e   Reference Page: 1336

Rationale: Stress urinary incontinence is thought to be most commonly caused by urethral hypermobility with loss of transmission of abdominal pressure to the proximal and mid-urethra. However, recent reports suggest an active mechanism involving compression of the urethra against the pubic symphysis maintains continence. Regardless of mechanism, vaginal suspension procedures, either suprapubic or vaginal approaches can be used to correct this problem resulting in a 50% to 90% cure rate. However, recognition of an intrinsic sphincter deficiency as an additional cause of urinary incontinence requires a different surgical procedure. Suspension procedures are much less effective for intrinsic sphincter problems. In this case, a pubovaginal fascial sling which compresses the outlet and prevents hypermobility corrects both problems. Alpha-adrenergic agonists and intravaginal estrogens may improve incontinence to a small degree, but do not represent treatments of choice for a combined defect.

27

Inflammatory Diseases of the Bladder

Grannum R. Sant

1. **A 30-year-old, sexually active woman is referred by her gynecologist because of recurrent episodes of cystitis. These occur 4 to 6 times a year associated with positive urine cultures for E. coli. The patient has no symptoms of flank pain or fever and her past urologic history is negative. Initial management should be:**

    a.   intravenous urogram and cystoscopy.
    b.   urethral dilatation.
    c.   voiding cystourethrogram.
    d.   low dose, long-term oral antimicrobial prophylaxis.
    e.   intravaginal estrogen therapy.

Correct Answer: d   Reference Page: 1331

Rationale: Recurrent bacterial cystitis in young women of reproductive age is due to bacterial reinfection. The reservoir for the bacteria is the vaginal introitus which allows uropathogenic bacteria from the lower gastrointestinal tract to adhere to its epithelial cells. Bacterial adherence is due to an inherited predisposition although sexual intercourse, diaphragm use, and spermicidals are additional risk factors.

As the lower urinary tract is normal in the majority of women with recurrent cystitis, there is no need for radiologic imaging, dilatation or cystoscopy. Antimicrobial prophylaxis (e.g., nightly or after intercourse) is recommended for treatment in young women. However, postmenopausal women with recurrent cystitis can be treated with topical estrogen applied to the vagina. This affects commensal lactobacilli in the vagina, lowers the pH and reduces the risk of reinfection.

2. **A 68-year-old man developed paraplegia following surgery for a spinal tumor. He was initially managed with clean intermittent catheterization and two months postoperatively, he was transferred to a nursing home. Indwelling Foley catheter (20F, 5 cc balloon) drainage was instituted. Six months later the patient is referred for urologic consultation because of persistent asymptomatic bacteriuria in spite of treatment with multiple courses of culture-specific antibiotics. Appropriate urologic treatment is:**

    a.   systemic, oral fluoroquinolone antimicrobial prophylaxis.
    b.   change to hydrophilic Foley catheter.
    c.   daily cleansing of the urethral meatus with antibiotic ointments.
    d.   transurethral prostatic resection and discontinuation of Foley.
    e.   nontreatment of asymptomatic bacteriuria.

Correct Answer: e   Reference Page: 1333

Rationale: Catheter-associated urinary tract infections are common in institutional-ized, elderly patients. Periurethral bacterial migration and the development of a bacterial biofilm on the catheter surface are the major causes of catheter-associated infections. Systemic antimicrobial therapy, daily meatal cleaning and use of hydrophilic catheters do not significantly reduce the risk of bacteriuria in patients with indwelling catheters. Transurethral prostatic resection in a paraplegic does not guarantee spontaneous voiding and discontinuation of Foley drainage. Asymptomatic bacteriuria in elderly, catheterized patients should not be treated with antibiotics, with the possible exception of bacteriuria due to urease-producing bacteriuria, e.g., Proteus, Pseudomonas, etc.

3. **Cyclophosphamide-induced hemorrhagic cystitis:**

   a. is due to the effect of N-acetyl cysteine on the bladder urothelium.
   b. can be prevented by Mesna (2-mercaptoethane sulfonate) and vigorous diuresis.
   c. is a surgical emergency requiring formalin bladder instillation under anesthesia.
   d. occurs in the majority of bone marrow transplant patients.
   e. is best treated by hyperbaric oxygen therapy.

   Correct Answer: b   Reference Page: 1337

   Rationale: The urotoxicity of cyclophosphamide (and other oxaza-phosphorine alkylating drugs) is due to the liver metabolite, acrolein. N-acetyl cysteine and 2-mercaptoethane sulfonate (Mesna) bind to the carbon double-bonds of acrolein to form non-toxic thioesters.

   The use of Mesna, vigorous hydration and an indwelling Foley catheter significantly reduces the risk of development of cyclophosphamide-induced hemorrhagic cystitis. If conservative measures (e.g., alum irrigation, prostaglandins, etc.) fail, formalin instillation under anesthesia may be necessary. Hyperbaric oxygen treatment is useful for radiation-induced hemorrhagic cystitis.

4. **Urologic consultation is obtained for a 28-year-old woman with a 3-year history of frequency, nocturia, vague pelvic pain and occasional dyspareunia. Gyneco-logic evaluation has been negative and multiple urine cultures revealed no significant bacteriuria. Urinalysis shows 0-2 WBC/bpf. The most likely diagnosis is:**

   a. pelvic and bladder endometriosis.
   b. the urethral syndrome.
   c. chronic interstitial cystitis.
   d. trichomonas vaginitis.
   e. urethral meatal stenosis.

Correct Answer: c   Reference Page: 1342

Rationale: Women with irritative voiding symptoms and pain (pelvic, vaginal) should be evaluated for chronic interstitial cystitis. The normal urinalysis effectively excludes the "urethral syndrome" (usually associated with pyuria $\pm$ low count bacteriuria) and vaginitis as possible diagnoses.

Empiric urethral dilatations have been done in the past to treat women with irritative voiding symptoms. There is no evidence that urethral stenosis contributes to the pathogenesis of these symptoms. Pelvic endometriosis is typically characterized by significant pelvic pain. However, some patients have chronic interstitial cystitis and coexistent endometriosis.

5.   **The diagnosis of interstitial cystitis is best made by:**

   a.   cystoscopy under anesthesia with bladder hydrodilatation.
   b.   bladder biopsy findings.
   c.   videourodynamic evaluation.
   d.   urine culture and cytology.
   e.   careful history and physical examination.

Correct Answer: a   Reference Page: 1343

Rationale: Interstitial cystitis is reliably diagnosed by cystoscopic evaluation under anesthesia with bladder hydrodilatation. The presence of glomerulations (dilated submucosal capillaries), submucosal hemorrhage or Hunner's ulcers (rare) confirm the diagnosis. Most patients with interstitial cystitis have normal bladder capacities under anesthesia. Urine culture and cytology are useful tests to exclude other pathology, e.g., infection, cancer, etc. However, negative culture/cytology findings are not confirmatory for diagnosis of interstitial cystitis. Radiologic imaging and videourodynamics are not essential components in the work-up of patients with suspected interstitial cystitis.

6.   **Urinary tract infections (UTIs) develop as a result of the interplay between bacterial pathogenicity and intrinsic host defenses. Which of the following statements is false?**

   a.   Bacterial adherence is an insignificant virulence mechanism.
   b.   Efficient bladder emptying prevents UTIs.
   c.   Prostatic antibacterial factors reduce the risk of UTIs in men.
   d.   Systemic disease and immunosuppression reduce host defenses.
   e.   The diaphragm is an acquired risk factor for UTIs in women.

Correct Answer: a   Reference Page: 1328

Rationale: Uropathogenic bacteria tend to have multiple bacterial adherence properties, e.g., fimbriae, etc. that allow attachment to epithelial surfaces. The body has a number of intrinsic defense mechanisms that prevent uropathogenic bacteria from causing UTIs.

Efficient voiding and lack of large post-void residual volumes are major defenses. When impaired, e.g., in bladder outlet obstruction secondary to BPH or in spinal cord injury, patients are at increased risk for UTIs. Furthermore, prostatic fluid is highly bactericidal and this partially explains the low prevalence of UTIs in non-elderly men. Acquired risk factors include systemic disease, immunosuppression, use of the diaphragm, etc.

7. **Malacoplakia is an uncommon, granulomatous disease of the genitourinary tract. Which of the following statements regarding malacoplakia is true?**

   a. Malacoplakia is a premalignant condition.
   b. Michaelis-Gutmann bodies occur in lymphocytes.
   c. Malacoplakia can be treated with Bethanechol.
   d. Malacoplakia never affects the upper urinary tract.
   e. It is never associated with urinary tract infections.

Correct Answer: c   Reference Page: 1336

Rationale: Malacoplakia is an uncommon genitourinary disease characterized by irritative voiding symptoms. It is a benign condition and felt to be due to incomplete phagocytosis and digestion of bacteria by histocytes. The typical Michaelis-Gutmann bodies are rounded intracytoplasmic inclusions ("owls-eyes") in large, eosinophilic histocytes.

Bethanechol increases intracellular cGMP which promotes phagocytosis of ingested bacteria. Antibiotics are usually employed in the treatment of malacoplakia because most patients have a history of recurrent UTIs. Malacoplakia can affect the entire genitourinary tract.

28
Urinary Fistulas
Kevin T. McVary

1.   **A healthy 36-year-old female is referred to your office from her obstetrician with complaints of total urinary incontinence. She is 3 weeks status postcesarean delivery. She is otherwise free of complaints except for the constant wetting from her vagina. She reports voiding normally with a reasonable urinary stream despite the incontinence. The urinalysis and urine culture done in your office are unremarkable. Cystoscopy and vaginoscopy done in the office reveal a relatively straightforward urinary fistula demonstrable in the midline near the posterior aspect of the bladder, well away from the ureteral orifices. Chromogen dye placed in the bladder at the time of your evaluation is noted to stain vaginal tampons consistent with a vesicovaginal fistula. An IVP shows prompt excretion of contrast on the left side while the right side shows delayed function and a mild hydronephrosis. The next best test to be performed is the following:**

a. CT scan with and without contrast to the pelvic region.
b. fulguration of the fistula tract.
c. a triple dye test.
d. retrograde ureterography.
e. abdominal exploration and consideration for a resection of the diagnosed vesicovaginal fistula with omental interposition.

Correct Answer: d   Reference Page: 1356

Rationale: Retrograde ureterography is the next best test to be performed on this patient. It is important to rule out additional causes of urinary fistula other than the already diagnosed vesicovaginal fistula. It is possible that the hydronephrosis is related to a ureteral injury or perhaps communication to the vagina itself. Retrograde ureterography will help you ascertain that. A diligent search should be made for any additional communications since many treatment failures have occurred in the past because less obvious fistulas were overlooked.

2.   **A 70-year-old female with multiple medical problems presents with a 1 mm fistula 1 week postoperatively. The best treatment for this individual should be:**

a. a transabdominal repair.
b. vaginal repair.
c. cystoscopic fulguration and catheter drainage.
d. Foley catheter drainage for 4-6 weeks.
e. wait 3 months for surgery.

Correct Answer: c   Reference Page: 1357

Rationale: In a 1 mm fistula noted soon after surgery, fulguration, catheter drainage and observation constitute the preferred management. The small size of the fistula also supports this approach. Transvaginal or transvesical repair is certainly ill advised given the time frame. Urinary diversion through catheter drainage would be the most conservative and one which could allow spontaneous healing to occur.

3. **A 35-year-old female has a large fistula at the bladder neck as well as a fistula near the right ureteral orifice. Duration of the fistula is greater than 6 months and is presumed secondary to a transvaginal hysterectomy. She has no radiation exposure. The best approach at operative management in this case is with:**

    a. a combined transvesical and transabdominal omental interposition.
    b. a transvaginal approach.
    c. urinary diversion.
    d. Foley catheter drainage.
    e. biopsy.

Correct Answer: a   Reference Page: 1358

Rationale: In this individual the combination of a large fistula at the bladder neck combined with a fistula near the ureteral orifice makes this a complex fistula (other complex fistulas include multiple fistulas near ureteral orifices or those induced by radiation). These complex cases are best approached transabdominally for: (1) better exposure, (2) acquiring adequate blood supply for the interposition of tissues (omentum), and (3) decreasing the chance of ureteral injury during repair.

4. **In freeing the omentum for interposition needs during fistula repair it is important to preserve the blood supply from the:**

    a. middle colic artery.
    b. gastroepiploic artery.
    c. gastroduodenal artery.
    d. superior mesenteric artery.
    e. pancreaticoduodenal artery.

Correct Answer: b   Reference Pages: 1360-1361

Rationale: Maximum mobilization of the omentum for use in pelvic reconstructive procedures is useful to seal off various areas, add blood supply, and provide better lymphatic drainage. It can be mobilized from right to left or from left to right depending on the operative needs. This sometimes requires mobilizing the omentum off the greater curvature of the stomach keeping the gastroepiploic vessels on the omentum and thus using this for the blood supply.

5. **A 55-year-old male with a history of colon carcinoma treated with pre- and postoperative radiation therapy required an indwelling ureteral stent for ureteral**

stenosis. He presents to the emergency room with copious bright red blood bleeding from a Foley catheter and hypotension responsive to fluid resuscitation. The next best step is:

a. arteriography.
b. immediate laparotomy.
c. remove the stent.
d. CT scan of the abdomen.
e. cystoscopy to localize the bleeding.

Correct Answer: b   Reference Pages: 1364-1365

Rationale: The finding of brisk bleeding from the urinary tract in a patient with radiation surgery, history of carcinoma, chemotherapy and in the presence of indwelling ureteral stents generally indicates a ureteral arterial fistula and immediate surgical exploration.

6.   **The most useful and sensitive study to establish the diagnosis of an enterovesical fistula is:**

a. barium enema.
b. cystogram.
c. CT scan.
d. cystoscopy.
e. po administration of charcoal.

Correct Answer: d   Reference Page:

Rationale: A high index of suspicion is essential for making a diagnosis of vesico-enteric fistula. Cystoscopy remains the most reliable diagnostic test with the presence of a localized area of edema or congestion being the typical finding in an early stage fistula. Cystoscopy also rules out other causes in the differential diagnosis and permits biopsy of the fistula. Cystography is the most useful radiologic examination with the "herald sign" seen best in the oblique views. Barium enema, flexible sigmoidoscopy, colonoscopy, rarely reveal the fistula. CT scan can reveal abnormalities suggesting a fistula but rarely shows the fistula itself. Whether or not magnetic resonance imaging improves the diagnostic sensitivity is unknown.

7.   **A 65-year-old female presents with a history of a radiation induced urethral vaginal fistula. Her history is also remarkable for ovarian carcinoma treated via laparotomy and resection of the omentum. In planning her operative repair the best choice of materials for interposition is:**

a.   labial fat pad.
b.   peritoneal flap brought out through the vaginal cuff.
c.   synthetic graft material.
d.   de-epithelialized segment of small bowel brought out through the vaginal cuff.
e.   gracilis muscle flaps.

Correct Answer: e   Reference Page: 1373
Rationale: Gracilis muscle flaps requires additional planning but the advantages include limited exposure to previous irradiation, ease of flap rotation below the genitourinary diaphragm, avoidance of intra-abdominal exposure.

29
Urothelial Tumors of the Bladder, Upper Tracts, and Prostate

M'Liss A. Hudson and William J. Catalona

1. **The most common environmental risk factor with the strongest association for the subsequent development of bladder cancer is:**

    a. coffee.
    b. cigarette smoke.
    c. phenacetin use.
    d. pelvic irradiation.
    e. artificial sweetener use.

    Correct Answer: b   Reference Pages: 1380-1382
    Rationale: Cigarette smoking is reported to cause bladder cancer in 25% to 60% of cases in industrialized countries. Coffee and artificial sweeteners have only weak relationships to subsequent bladder tumor development. Exposure to pelvic irradiation is infrequent in the general population. Phenacetin use is banned in the U.S. and its use limited in most countries, so exposure to phenacetin is also infrequent.

2. **A mucosal lesion frequently found in association with invasive transitional cell carcinoma of the bladder which may be a precursor lesion to muscle invasive cancer is:**

    a. squamous metaplasia.
    b. nephrogenic adenoma.
    c. cystitis glandularis.
    d. Von Brunn's nests.
    e. carcinoma in situ.

    Correct Answer: e   Reference Pages: 1384-1387
    Rationale: Carcinoma in situ is composed of highly anaplastic cells limited to the mucosa of the bladder. Forty-two percent to 83% of patients with carcinoma in situ ultimately develop invasive bladder cancer. Cystitis glandularis (intestinal-type) may be a precursor of adenocarcinoma of the bladder. The other lesions are all benign.

3.   **The stage of bladder cancer with the best prognosis is:**

    a.   carcinoma in situ (pTis).
    b.   papillary mucosally-confined tumor (pTa).
    c.   papillary lamina propria invasive tumor (pT_1).
    d.   superficial muscle-invasive tumor (pT_2)
    e.   metastatic tumor (pT_4).

Correct Answer: b   Reference Pages: 1400-1402
Rationale: Five-year survival rates are 95% for pTa tumors, but only 72% to 82% for pTis and pT_1 disease, 64% for pT_2, and 25% for pT_4 tumors.

4.   **The p53 tumor suppressor gene is:**

    a.   not found in bladder cancer.
    b.   associated with a low risk for tumor progression.
    c.   a poor prognostic factor associated with a high risk for tumor progression.
    d.   activated by tryptophan metabolites.
    e.   found on X-chromosomes.

Correct Answer: c   Reference Page: 1403
Rationale: Several independent studies have shown that the p53 suppressor gene is a poor prognostic factor in bladder cancer. It has been found to predict progression to muscle-invasive cancer in patients with pTis, pTa, and pT_1 tumors.

5.   **The most common side effect of intravesical Bacillus Calmette-Guerin (BCG) therapy is:**

    a.   gross hematuria.
    b.   fever.
    c.   arthralgias.
    d.   irritative voiding symptoms.
    e.   malaise.

Correct Answer: d   Reference Page: 1413
Rationale: Eighty percent of patients treated with intravesical BCG therapy experience irritative voiding symptoms. Fever, arthralgias, malaise, and gross hematuria occur in fewer than 30% of patients so treated.

6. **All of the following are relative contraindications to performing a partial cystectomy for invasive bladder cancer except:**

   a. diffuse carcinoma in situ.
   b. extension of cancer into the trigone and bladder neck.
   c. recurrent multifocal disease.
   d. urachal adenocarcinoma.
   e. encroachment of tumor on a ureteral orifice.

Correct Answer: d   Reference Pages: 1417-1418, 1392

Rationale: The best candidate for a partial cystectomy is a patient with a solitary, primary tumor which can be resected with a 2 cm margin without encroachment on a ureteral orifice or the bladder neck. The presence of carcinoma in situ, recurrent multifocal disease, extension of disease into the trigone or bladder neck often preclude obtaining a tumor-free margin when a partial cystectomy is attempted. Encroachment on a ureteral orifice is a relative contraindication since the ureter may be reimplanted if necessary to obtain a 2 cm margin.

7. **The most effective chemotherapeutic regimens for the treatment of metastatic bladder cancer usually include which agent?**

   a. Actinomycin D
   b. Thiotepa
   c. Bleomycin
   d. Cis-platinum
   e. Streptozocin

Correct Answer: d   Reference Pages: 1431-1432

Rationale: The most effective chemotherapeutic regimens are M-VAC, CMV, and CISCA, all of which contain cis-platinum.

8. **The most common type of bladder cancer in children is:**

   a. lymphoma.
   b. pheochromocytoma.
   c. neurofibroma.
   d. transitional cell carcinoma.
   e. rhabdomyosarcoma.

Correct Answer: e   Reference Pages: 1434-1435

Rationale: Embryonal rhabdomyosarcomas (sarcoma botryoides) usually arise on the trigone of the bladder and are the most common tumor in the pediatric age group.

30
Urinary Diversion and Continent Reservoir

Joseph G. Trapasso

1. **Relative contraindications in performing a ureterosigmoidostomy include all** *except*:

   a. prior large bowel disease or dilated ureters.
   b. renal or hepatic impairment.
   c. pelvic irradiation.
   d. short bowel syndrome.
   e. anal sphincteric dysfunction.

   Correct Answer: d   Reference Page: 1466, 1497
   Rationale: Due to the significant potential for associated metabolic, anastomotic and continence problems postoperatively, ureterosigmoidostomy in such patients should be avoided.

2. **In patients with ureterosigmoidostomy, recommended follow-up investigations include all** *except*:

   a. intravenous pyelogram.
   b. serum electrolytes.
   c. barium enema.
   d. stool for occult blood.
   e. colonoscopy.

   Correct Answer: c   Reference Page: 1468
   Rationale: Barium enemas are relatively contraindicated because of the potential of reflux of this material in causing associated septic events.

3. **The preferred method of urinary diversion in the patient with previous abdominal/pelvic radiation is the:**

   a. ileal conduit.
   b. jejunal conduit.
   c. transverse colon conduit.
   d. ureterosigmoidostomy.
   e. sigmoid colon conduit.

   Correct Answer: c   Reference Page: 1475
   Rationale: In most instances, the transverse colon resides outside the field of pelvic and lower abdominal radiation.

4.   **Electrolyte/metabolic abnormalities resulting from jejunal interposition for urinary diversion include all *except*:**

a.   hypermagnesemia.
b.   hyponatremia.
c.   hypercalcemia.
d.   acidosis.
e.   hypochloremia.

Correct Answer: a   Reference Page: 1496

Rationale: Electrolyte/metabolic abnormalities in jejunal conduits result from excessive secretion of sodium chloride coupled with an increased reabsorption of potassium and hydrogen ions.

5.   **In continent reservoir construction, detubularization of the intended bowel segment provides:**

a.   better compliance.
b.   improved continence.
c.   less reflux.
d.   decreased pressure.
e.   less stone formation.

Correct Answer: d   Reference Page: 1477

Rationale: Antimesenteric disruption of the circular smooth musculature of the bowel segment(s) reduces the risk of high-pressure contractions seen in intact, undisrupted portions of continent urinary diversions.

6.   **A 65-year-old man with a ureterosigmoidostomy and chronic acidosis with serum bicarbonate levels in the 10-15 mM/l range also has congestive heart failure and heart disease. The best treatment for his acidosis is:**

a.   citrate.
b.   bicarbonate.
c.   nicotinic acid.
d.   Bicitra.
e.   potassium citrate.

Correct Answer: c   Reference Page: 1496

Rationale: Most medications effective in correction of metabolic acidosis possess a substantial sodium content which may exacerbate existing cardiac or renal disease.

7. **The continence mechanism of continent cutaneous catheterizable urinary reservoirs such as the Indiana pouch rely on the:**

    a. detubularization of the bowel segments.
    b. intact ileocecal valve.
    c. tapered efferent limb.
    d. buttressed efferent limb.
    e. intussuscepted and stapled ileal segment.

Correct Answer: b   Reference Page: 1492

Rationale: Pressure studies have indicated that the nascent ileocecal valve is the primary structure involved in maintaining continence in reservoirs such as the Indiana pouch.

8. **The incidence of prolonged urinary-intestinal anastomotic extravasation has been reduced by:**

    a. bowel detubularization.
    b. use of antirefluxing anastomotic techniques.
    c. monofilament absorbable suture.
    d. meticulous dissection with preservation of periureteral vasculature.
    e. ureteral stents/catheters.

Correct Answer: e   Reference Page: 1472

Rationale: The routine use of ureteral stents/catheters has reduced the incidence of persistent or prolonged urine extravasation from the site of the ureterointestinal anastomosis to less than 5%.

31
Benign Prostatic Hyperplasia

John T. Grayhack

1.   **The symptoms of voiding dysfunction associated with the presence of BPH:**

     a.   include terminal dribbling as a prominent characteristic component.

     b.   can be diagnosed on the basis of a characteristic symptom complex.

     c.   increase progressively in prevalence in men as they age in contrast to a much lower prevalence in women as they age.

     d.   shows a proportional increase in incidence, prevalence, and severity relating to the size of the adenomatous growth.

     e.   are not either persistent or progressive in at least one-third of the men in whom they are recognized.

Correct Answer: e   Reference Page: 1529, 1530, 1535

Rationale: The symptom complex designated "prostatism" to indicate its relationship to BPH voiding dysfunction is neither specific for men with BPH nor clearly related to the size of the enlarged prostate. The symptoms are shared among others by aging women. Terminal dribbling occurs at all ages. Symptoms may raise the question of BPH voiding dysfunction; they do not establish the diagnosis. Symptom status and objective measures of voiding often are not closely correlated. Observations of control groups in drug studies and of longitudinally observed men indicate that voiding symptoms thought to be secondary to be BPH have improved or stabilized in a sizable percentage of men with time.

2.   **Acute urinary retention in men:**

     a.   has been shown to be associated with increased levels of Actin, Myosin, and hydroxyproline in the urine.

     b.   is significantly increased in men with marked hesitancy and intermittency.

     c.   is almost certain to be followed by symptoms and objective findings supporting the need for therapeutic intervention.

     d.   may be a sequelae of prostatic infarction.

     e.   is likely to respond promptly to initiation of 5 alpha reductase inhibitor therapy.

Correct Answer: d   Reference Page: 1535, 1536

Rationale: Development of acute urinary retention is unpredictable in men with BPH and is apparently induced at times by develoment of a prostatic infarct. A limited group of men without incident related or identifiable ancillary cause for the episode of acute retention are able to void after catheterization and have prolonged periods with limited symptoms. Finasteride therapy requires months to achieve a significant mass reduction and would not be expected to help achieve spontaneous voiding in individuals in acute retention. No urinary studies reporting biochemical evidence of muscle damage in pateints with acute retention are known to me.

3. **With regard to anatomic BPH:**

a. histologic evidence of BPH in a given age group is much more common in the United States and western European inhabitants than in Japanese living in Japan.
b. is predominantly a cellular proliferative disease, ultimately producing recognizable gross changes in about half or less of the patients with histologic disease.
c. is characterized histologically by absence of the acinar basal cell layer.
d. in contrast to the so-called surgical capsule or compressed peripheral zone tissue is devoid of alpha adrenergic receptors.
e. has a relative and absolute decrease in stromal components compared to normal prostate.

Correct Answer: b   Reference Page: 1509, 1515, 1516, 1519, 1521, 1534

Rationale: Histologic BPH has a similar prevalence increasing with age in all geographic and racial groups studied. Gross BPH, the clinically important lesion, is eventually recognizable in half or fewer of the patients with histologic BPH in the United States. BPH has alpha adrenergic receptors and has an absolute increase in all stromal components including smooth muscle compared to the normal prostate. The acini of BPH has a definite basal cell layer; the absence of a basal cell layer seen in carcinoma. Stromal components account for an increasing percentage of BPH tissue compared to the normal prostate.

4. **Patients undergoing transurethral resection of the prostate:**

a. for moderate symptoms are significantly more likely to avoid management failure and experience improved symptoms than those electing watchful waiting.
b. have an establisehd prolonged increased risk of developing serious de novo cardiovascular disease in patients subjected to open prostatectomy.
c. rarely will experience reversal of symptoms of urgency or urgency incontinence associated with BPH.
d. may develop severe hyponatremia that almost always requires prompt administration of a diuretic and hypertonic saline.
e. currently usually are free of other significant illnesses, accounting for the current low mortality.

Correct Answer: a   Reference Page: 1550, 1557, 1559
Rationale: A prospective VA study has demonstrated that TURP affords less risk of treatment failure and improved symptomatic status compared to watchful waiting in men with moderate urinary symptoms. The symptoms of urgency and urgency incontinence associated with BPH have been reported to be common, although not always reversible. Hypertonic saline is a useful therapeutic tool to treat severe postTURP hyponatremia but is rarely required. The low operative and perioperative mortality following TURP is achieved despite significant comorbidity. The suggestion that TURP leads to long-term increased risk of developing fatal cardiovascular disease has not been supported by accumulating evidence.

5. **With regard to the use of drug therapy to treat BPH related voiding problems:**

   a. both alpha adrenergic blockers and 5 alpha reductase inhibitors have an appreciable risk of serious side effects.
   b. the response of alpha adrenergic blockers and 5 alpha reductase inhibitors is usually prompt or lacking.
   c. the immediate effect of alpha adrenergic blockers on flow rate approximates the results achieved with TURP and has been demonstrated to be durable.
   d. antiandrogen therapy may control recurrent prostatic bleeding.
   e. alpha adrenergic blockers and 5 alpha reductase inhibitors have clearly altered long-term natural history of BPH voiding dysfunction.

Correct Answer: d   Reference Page: 1535, 1537, 1538
Rationale: Antiandrogen therapy is effective therapy in many patients with recurrent hematuria due to BPH. The voiding response to alpha adrenergic blockers is usually prompt but is delayed to 5 alpha reductase inhibitors. Side effects from these drugs have been limited in frequency and severity but their effect on the long-term course of BPH and its associated voiding dysfunction has not been established. The symptomatic and urodynamic effects of TURP are markedly better than those achieved with drug therapy.

6. **The advantages of laser prostatectomy compared to TURP are:**

   a. the production of a more controlled tissue destructive process resulting in more effective ablation of BPH tissue.
   b. the earlier achievement of a catheter free state.
   c. the ability to control bleeding even in patients on anticoagulant therapy.
   d. the procedure usually can be carried out under sedation and local anesthesia.
   e. retrograde ejaculation does not occur.

Correct Answer: c   Reference Page: 1561-1562

Rationale: Laser prostatectomy has achieved satisfactory voiding results in limited reported trials. This is accomplished with minimal blood loss even in patients on anticoagulants. Regional or general anesthesia comparable to surgical excision procedures is usually required for laser prostatectomy. Prolonged catheter drainage is necessary in a significant cohort of the patients undergoing laser prostatectomy.

7.   **The normal prostate:**

a.   is separated into ventral (fibromuscular) and dorsal (glandular) regions by the urethra that courses in a gentle slope from the bladder neck through the verumontanum.

b.   has a so-called capsule that is actually a condensation of stromal elements that is incomplete at the apex.

c.   has urethral branches of the prostatovesicular artery that almost invariably enter the bladder neck at 5 and 7 o'clock.

d.   has neurovascular bundles supplying the prostate and containing the penile corporal nerves that lie midway between the ventral and dorsal aspects of the prostate.

e.   has the major prostatic ducts terminating linearly along the course of the urethra.

Correct Answer: b   Reference Page: 1501, 1503, 1504, 1505

Rationale: The so-called capsule of the prostate is actually a condensation of stromal elements, not a true capsule; it is described as incomplete at the apex. It, therefore has continuity with the internal architecture of the prosate. The neurovascular bundle is located at the posterior lateral boundary of the prostate. The blood supply at the bladder neck usually but not invariably enters the prosate at 5 and 7 o'clock. The major prostatic ducts terminate adjacent or distal to the verumontanum. The urethra has an angular course in the mid-urethra.

8.   **The adult human prostate:**

a.   has in contrast to BPH more epithelial than any other tissue on stereological assessment.

b.   has striated as well as smooth muscle throughout the glandular structure.

c.   has a high concentration of the enzyme 5 alpha reductase, type II, in the stromal and basal cells but little or none in the epithelial cells.

d.   has a high concentration of citric acid in its secretion, a probable major factor in controlling bacterial prostatic infection.

e.   has a prominent prostatic growth factor, basic fibroblast growth factor (bFGF), that functions primarily as a prostatic epithelial cell stimulant.

Correct Answer: c   Reference Page: 1507, 1512, 1514, 1515, 1517
Rationale: Surprisingly the enzyme 5 alpha reductase type II is not demonstrable by histochemical techniques in the epithelial cells of the prostate but is in stromal and basal cells. The finding brings into question the classical concept of androgen stimulation of prostate proliferation. Stromal elements predominate in normal prostate and BPH. Striated muscle is normally present in the anterior and anterolateral aspects of the gland, not throughout it. Basic FGF is a stromal stimulant and zinc, not citrate, also present in very high concentration in the prostatic fluid, is thought to be important in controlling bacterial prostatic infections.

9.   **BPH:**

   a.   almost never produces renal failure in the absence of markedly increased prostatic mass.
   b.   is comparably reduced in mass by balloon dilatation, finasteride and transrectal wave therapy.
   c.   has a significantly increased concentration of dihydrotestosterone (DHT) compared to the peripheral prostate.
   d.   undergoes significant tissue necrosis when subjected to temperatures of 42° to 44° C for 1 minute or more.
   e.   develops a significant increase in tissue testosterone concentration with finasteride therapy in some men.

Correct Answer: e   Reference Page: 1523, 1529, 1538, 1561, 1563
Rationale: BPH and the peripheral prostate have comparable concentrations of DHT. Finasteride causes a marked reduction in DHT concentration but the tissue testosterone levels are significantly increased. No significant reduction in prostatic mass is produced by balloon dilatation or transrectal wave therapy. Tissue temperatures exceeding 44° C are necessary to produce tissue necrosis of normal as contrasted to temperature sensitive malignant cells. The effects of BPH on voiding are not directly correlated with prostatic mass.

10.   **Open (suprapubic, retropubic, perineal) prostatectomy:**

   a.   is followed by impotence in the majority of patients.
   b.   usually results in an excellent symptomatic improvement.
   c.   has a higher incidence of postoperative incontinence than TURP.
   d.   almost never (less than 0.3%) requires a subsequent procedure for treatment of BPH.
   e.   is rarely associated with retrograde ejaculation.

Correct Answer: b   Reference Page: 1556, 1558
Rationale: The BPH guidelines report indicate that symptomatic improvement following open prostatectomy occurs in the highest percentage of treated patients reported. Although retrograde ejaculation occurs in most patients, potency was preserved in most (80%+) patients and the postoperative incontinence rate was lower than for TURP. Selected current individual series, as contrasted to the data analyzed for the guidelines review, indicate a low requirement for blood transfusion and low risk of mortality but a surprising persistent need for regeneration in a small group of patients.

11. **With regard to the complications that follow TURP or open prostatectomy:**

   a. evidence suggests that prolonged antibiotic administration has no effect on the incidence of postoperative urethral stricture.
   b. problem postoperative bleeding is usually best controlled by combining catheter manipulation and administration of appropriate coagulation enhancing drugs.
   c. postoperative bacteremia is almost always signaled by clinical symptoms.
   d. absorption of an appropriately constituted irrigating fluid such as glycine may have systemic metabolic as well as dilutional effects.
   e. postoperative urinary incontinence is avoidable if the visually identifiable external sphincter is preserved.

Correct Answer: d   Reference Page: 1540, 1547, 1548, 1549, 1550
Rationale: Absorbed glycine may be metabolized to produce free ammonia contributing to a variety of neurologic symptoms. Bacteremia is much more common than septicemia in patients subjected to TURP. The extent of essential functional components of the external sphincter is not limited to the visually identifiable sphincter area. Problem postoperative TURP bleeding is best managed by a systematic effort to identify and control specific causes. Evidence has recently been presented that suggests prolonged antibiotic administration may reduce the incidence of postoperative strictures.

12.   **The voiding dysfunction associated with BPH may:**

a.   be relieved by incision of the prostatic capsule without removing prostatic mass.
b.   is classically, but not always, associated with normal intravesical pressure accompanied by poor urinary flow.
c.   is accompanied by increased muscular and decreased connective tissue mass in the bladder.
d.   is almost always associated with normal bladder compliance, despite the anatomic and physiologic changes induced by BPH.
e.   Often accompanied by the development of trabeculation in the bladder in anatomical manifestation of the increased smooth muscle.

Correct Answer: a   Reference Page: 1529, 1530, 1534, 1546
Rationale: Both endoscopic (TUIP) and open capsular incision have produced symptomatic and urodynamic improvement in BPH voiding dysfunction without removing prostatic mass. The relative increase in connective tissue is greater than in the muscular tissue in the bladder of elderly patients. Classically, the resting tone and voiding pressure are higher than normal and the flow rate lower than normal in patients with BPH voiding dysfunction. Bladder compliance is ultimately compromised by the tissue changes noted. The tissue making up the visual trabecular pattern is primarily connective tissue.

32
Carcinoma of the Prostate
James M. Kozlowski and John T. Grayhack

1. **All the following statements regarding prostatic intraepithelial neoplasia (PIN) are true *except*:**

   a. three grades or subsets of PIN are currently recognized.
   b. disruptions of the basal cell layer may occur in grade III PIN.
   c. PIN is most often associated with peripheral zone cancers.
   d. needle aspiration cytology can distinguish high-grade PIN and invasive cancer.
   e. PIN may be associated with elevated levels of PSA.

   Correct Answer: d   Reference Page: 1586
   Rationale: The histologic features typically demonstrated in grade III PIN include: (1) a cribriform-like acinar architecture, (2) disruption of the basal cell layer in 56% of cases, (3) markedly enlarged nuclei displaying an increased chromatin pattern, and (4) the frequent presence of large pleomorphic nucleoli. Invasive cancers will frequently demonstrate the latter two cytologic features. For this reason, aspiration cytology can not reliably distinguish these two conditions.

2. **Ductal cancers constitute the largest subset of atypical prostate adenocarcinomas. All of the following statements regarding ductal cancers are true *except*:**

   a. low columnar epithelium lines the primary/secondary ductal system of the prostate.
   b. endometrioid carcinomas are a variant of primary ductal adenocarcinomas.
   c. gross hematuria is a common presenting symptom.
   d. skeletal metastases associated with ductal cancers are usually osteoblastic.
   e. metastatic ductal carcinomas do not respond to androgen deprivation therapy.

   Correct Answer: e   Reference Page: 1593
   Rationale: Primary and secondary ductal tumors constitute about 3% of prostate cancers and appear to arise following malignant degeneration of low columnar epithelium lining primary, secondary, or tertiary ducts. The present consensus is that so-called endometrioid carcinomas of the prostate represent a variant of primary ductal adenocarcinoma with endometrioid features. These tumors tend to be multicentric and demonstrate an aggressive phenotype with a proclivity for early stromal invasion. Due to their central location, gross hematuria is a frequent presenting symptom. Although conflicting information exists regarding the androgen dependency of these tumors, several studies have documented the presence of PAP and PSA in the majority of them. Skeletal metastases tend to be osteoblastic and are associated with elevations of blood markers. Most patients will respond to androgen deprivation therapy. As a

group, however, these patients tend to have a slightly worse prognosis when compared with those whose tumors arise from acinar elements.

3. **The anatomic information provided by transrectal ultrasonography (TRUS) regarding the prostate is superior to that obtained by either computed tomographic (CT) scanning or magnetic resonance imaging (MRI). All of the following statements regarding TRUS are true *except*:**

   a. The ultrasonographic appearance of the normal peripheral zone (PZ) is described as isoechoic.
   b. The normal central zone (CZ) is somewhat hypoechoic when compared with the PZ.
   c. There is no pathognomonic appearance of prostate cancer on TRUS.
   d. About 30% of prostate cancers originate from the central and transition zones.
   e. Hypoechoic foci may represent areas of acute inflammation, cysts, infarcts, small nodules of hyperplasia, blood vessels or muscle tissue.

Correct Answer: b   Reference Pages: 1599-1600
Rationale: The PZ constitutes 75% of the normal glandular volume and occupies the posterior, lateral, and apical regions. Its ultrasonographic appearance is described as isoechoic. The CZ is somewhat hyperechoic when compared with the PZ and constitutes the remaining 25% of glandular volume. All the other statements regarding TRUS are true.

4. **Staging is a clinical effort to identify the phase of the natural history of carcinoma of the prostate that exists in a patient by documenting the site and extent of tumor involvement. All the following staging designations for carcinoma of the prostate are correct *except*:**

   a. Stage T_{1c} tumors are unsuspected, organ-confined lesions detected because of an elevated PSA.
   b. T_{2b} tumors are organ-confined lesions which occupy more than half of a lobe, but not both lobes.
   c. Obliteration of both lateral sulci define stage T_{3a} tumors.
   d. Stage T_{2b} cancers involve the levator muscles or pelvic side wall.
   e. N1 disease involves one regional lymph node < to 1 cm.

Correct Answer: c   Reference Page: 1610
Rationale: Tumors that have demonstrated periprostatic extension on clinical examination but have no evidence of distal metastasis are classified as stage T_3, T_4. The 1992 UICC-AJCC classification separates unilateral (T_{3a}) and bilateral (T_{3b}) extracapsular extension and seminal vesical invasion (T_{2c})

5.   **Prostate specific antigen (PSA) is a serum protein belonging to the family of glandular kallikreins that is an androgen controlled secretory product of the prostate. All of the following statements regarding PSA are true *except*:**

a.   PSA is a lysosomal protein whose natural substrate is semenogelin.
b.   PSA may stimulate tumor growth by releasing insulin-like growth factors from their binding proteins.
c.   The in vivo half-life of PSA is 2.2 days.
d.   Lymph node and skeletal metastasis are unusual if the PSA is less than 10 ng/ml.
e.   PSA is a more sensitive tumor marker than prostatic acid phosphatase.

Correct Answer: a   Reference Pages: 1611-1612
Rationale: Unlike PAP which is a lysosomal enzyme, PSA is a cytoplasmic glycoprotein. The natural physiologic substrate for PSA is semenogelin which is the major protein of the seminal vesicle coagulum. Recent evidence suggest that PSA itself is a prostatic mitogen and that it may enhance the invasion of extracellular matrix in a manner similar to urokinase-type plasminogen activator which is another serine protease with which it shares sequence homology. Nondetectable levels of PSA should be noted within one month after a curative radical prostatectomy. The delayed recognition of a detectable increasing serum PSA in a post-radical prostatectomy patient indicates persistent carcinoma, and marker evidence may precede classical evidence of disease by as much as five years.

6.   **Radical prostatectomy is usually carried out in an attempt to cure carcinoma of the prostate. The goal is achieved with regularity in patients in whom the pathologic examination of the excised specimen reveals a tumor that has not escaped the anatomic confines of the gland. Recent observations indicate that tumor-free survival may also be enhanced in individuals in whom the extraprostatic disease is excised with a tumor-free margin, or perhaps in those with extra-prostatic tumor treated with adjunctive external radiation. All of the following statements regarding radical prostatectomy are true *except*:**

a.   The endopelvic fascia should be incised near the point of its reflection along the side wall of the pelvis.
b.   The puboprostatic ligaments constitute a pyramid-shaped structure that serves as a component of the urethral suspensory mechanism.
c.   The rectourethralis muscle is actually the posterior element of the striated urethral sphincter.
d.   Nerve-sparing should be abandoned when capsular penetration is suspected by the presence of fibrosis and induration.
e.   The perineal approach may have some potential advantages over the retropubic with regard to fewer positive surgical margins and lower complication rates.

Correct Answer: e   Reference Pages: 1645-1648

Rationale: Radical perineal prostatectomy has some potential advantages over the retropubic approach with respect to controlling blood loss, facilitating the urethrovesical anastomosis, and decreased postoperative pain. There is no difference in the incidence of positive surgical margins, nor is there any difference in short-term/long-term complication rates when the two approaches are compared. All the other statements regarding radical prostatectomy are true.

7. **All the following statements regarding radiation therapy are true *except*:**

   a. Neutrons and protons constitute heavy particle beams.
   b. The G_2 phase of the cell cycle is the most sensitive to radiation.
   c. Aneuploid prostate cancers tend to be radiation-resistant.
   d. Conformal treatment planning may permit a 10% to 20% dose increase without enhancing complications.
   e. Neoadjuvant hormonal therapy may enhance local tumor control.

Correct Answer: b   Reference Page: 1654

Rationale: It is now well established that double-strand breaks in the DNA molecule account for most radiation-induced cytotoxicity. The M phase and the boundary between G_1 and S phases are the most sensitive to radiation. All the other statements regarding therapy are correct.

8. **In 1941 Huggins and Hodges published their landmark observations establishing the efficacy of androgen-ablative/suppressive therapy for the treatment of patients with disseminated prostate cancer. This approach remains the cornerstone of therapy in patients with advanced-stage disease. All of the following statements regarding endocrine therapy are correct *except*:**

   a. A 95% reduction in serum testosterone is often achieved within three hours following castration.
   b. Both low-dose Megace and DES effectively control hot flashes.
   c. Flutamide and other anti-androgens may promote tumor growth in those prostate cancers with mutated androgen receptor genes.
   d. Complete androgen suppression is useful in all patients with metastatic prostate cancer.
   e. Intermittent endocrine therapy may delay the emergence of the androgen-independent phenotype.

Correct Answer: d   Reference Page: 1672

Rationale: Crawford and associates (1989) conducted a randomized, double-blind trial involving 603 men with previous untreated stage D_2 prostate cancer. Those randomized to receive both leuprolide plus flutamide exhibited a longer progression-free interval (16.5 vs 13.9 months; $p = .039$) and an increase in the median length of survival (35.6 vs 28.3 months; $p = .035$). It should be emphasized that improvement was most noteworthy in those patients with minimal disease, exhibiting a good performance status, and was particularly apparent during the first 12 weeks of treatment. Furthermore, in their analysis of progression-free survival, the authors chose to discount changes in the bone scan noted at the first three-month assessment. All the other statements regarding endocrine therapy are correct.

9. **About 75% of patients with metastatic carcinoma of the prostate demonstrate evidence of both objective and subjective improvement following the initiation of androgen-ablative therapy. The duration of benefit lasts from a few months to several years. The emergence of androgen-independent disease is an ominous sign since one half of these patients will succumb to the disease within the first year following relapse and most of the remainder will die as a result of the disease process or related causes within two years. All of the following statements regarding the systemic therapy of androgen-independent disease are correct *except*:**

a. The cytotoxic effects of estramustine are attributable to its disruption of microtubule assembly.
b. Suramin inhibits the binding of growth factors to their receptors, inhibits angiogenesis, and decreases cell motility.
c. Increased expression of the E-cadherin gene is associated with the androgen-independent phenotype.
d. Liarozole and phenylacetate are differentiation-inducing agents.
e. Tumor destruction by cytotoxic T-cells requires expression of tumor-associated antigens and class I MHC antigens.

Correct Answer: c   Reference Page: 1684

Rationale: Although the actual mechanisms associated with the emergence of the androgen-independent phenotype remain unclear, it appears that both genetic and epigenetic events may play a role in this phenomenon, which is typified by cellular dedifferentiation. The numerous adverse tumor cell features which have been associated with androgen-independent prostate cancers are delineated on page 1684. Note that these aggressive tumor systems are often associated with decreased tumor cell cohesiveness and increased invasiveness due to reduced expression of the E-cadherin gene. The latter is a transmembrane glycoprotein which plays an integral role in calcium-mediated cell-cell adhesion.

10. **Many recent studies have demonstrated that PSA is not secreted exclusively by the adluminal (secretory) cells of the prostate gland. Rather than being prostate-specific it appears that PSA is a rather ubiquitous molecule which may be synthesized/secreted by many tissues possessing steroid hormone receptors activated by an appropriate ligand (Yu and associates: Cancer Research, 55:1603-1606,1995). All of the following may constitute nonprostatic sources of PSA *except*:**

a. the urethral and anal glands of males and females.
b. 30% to 40% of female breast tumors.
c. tumors of the lung, colon, ovary, liver, kidney, adrenal, parotid, skin, and salivary glands.
d. normal endometrial tissue.
e. milk from lactating women.

Correct Answer: a   Reference Page: 1652

Rationale: All of these statements are correct with the exception of A. Nonprostatic sources of PSA have been identified in male and female urethral glands and the anal glands of the male (but not female). Of interest, PSA-producing breast tumors are associated with the presence of steroid hormone receptors and exhibit a more favorable overall prognosis. Although still somewhat speculative, it would appear that PSA may play an important regulatory role in normal breast tissue; fetal growth; insulin-like growth factor activity; osteoblast proliferation; the proteolytic modulation of cell adhesion receptors inducing the temporary contact-inhibition of tumor cells; and uterine function (Yu and associates: Cancer Research, 55: 1603-1606, 1995).

33
Prostatitis
Jackson E. Fowler, Jr.

1. **The most important historical clue to the cause of chronic prostatic symptomatology is the:**

    a. symptomatic response to antimicrobial therapy.
    b. severity of symptoms.
    c. symptomatic response to oxybutynin therapy.
    d. symptomatic response to doxazosin therapy.
    e. results from past urine cultures.

    Correct Answer: e   Reference Page: 1720

    Rationale: Urinary tract infections are infrequent in men but chronic bacterial prostatitis is always accompanied by bacteriuria. Therefore, a history of culture-documented urinary tract infections should alert the clinician to the possibility of chronic bacterial prostatitis. Conversely, if the urine cultures have been sterile during symptomatic episodes nonbacterial prostatitis or prostatodynia are the most likely diagnoses.

2. **A healthy 54-year-old man presents with fever, chills, and irritative voiding symptoms. The prostate is enlarged and tender and the urinalysis reveals numerous leukocytes and bacteria. Hospitalization does not appear to be warranted. The drug of choice for treatment of the infection is:**

    a. trimethoprim.
    b. trimethoprim-sulfamethoxazole.
    c. ciprofloxacin.
    d. carbenicillin.
    e. nitrofurantoin.

    Correct Answer: c   Reference Page: 1732

    Rationale: Ciprofloxicin, a fluoroquinolone antibiotic achieves high serum levels, has broad-spectrum antibacterial activities and is capable of eradicating infections of the prostate gland. Ciprofloxicin is particularly useful for the treatment of serious infections on an outpatient basis.

3.   **The treatment of choice for chronic prostatic symptomatology that is not accompanied by bacteriuria or by an increased density of leukocytes in the prostatic fluid is:**

a.   psychiatric counseling.
b.   transurethral thermal therapy.
c.   finasteride.
d.   doxazosin.
e.   prostatic massage.

Correct Answer: d   Reference Page: 1739

Rationale: An alpha adrenergic blockade with doxazosin reduces the smooth muscle tone in the bladder outlet and external sphincter and provides symptomatic relief in a majority of men with prostatodynia. The efficacy of prostatic heating is not well defined and prostatic massage is of symptomatic benefit in an occasional patient only. The 5-alpha reductase inhibitor finasteride is of potential but unproven benefit. Psychiatric counseling should be considered only when all other therapeutic measures have failed.

4.   **Kirby-Bauer antimicrobial susceptibility testing may underestimate the number of potentially useful antibiotics for the treatment of:**

a.   pyelonephritis.
b.   acute bacterial prostatitis.
c.   chronic bacterial prostatitis.
d.   bacteriuria.
e.   prostatodynia.

Correct Answer: d   Reference Page: 1730

Rationale: Kirby-Bauer susceptibility testing estimates the susceptibility of an infecting organism to drug concentrations that are achievable in the serum. However, most antibiotics are concentrated in the urine and achieve levels that are 100 to 1000 times greater than that in the serum. Since the infecting organisms in patients with bacteriuria are confined to the urine, the Kirby-Bauer test often underestimates the number of potentially useful antimicrobial treatments.

5.   A **72-year-old man with a PSA of 2.0 ng/ml is found to have a diffusely
indurated prostate gland. He had undergone a transurethral resection of the
prostate ten years earlier for histologically proven benign prostatic hyperplasia
and currently has no voiding symptoms or urinary tract infection. A prostate
biopsy reveals granulomatous prostatitis. The most appropriate management is:**

a.   suppressive antimicrobial therapy.
b.   an evaluation to rule out sarcoidosis.
c.   a repeat prostate biopsy in six months.
d.   observation.
e.   transurethral thermal therapy.

Correct Answer: d   Reference Page: 1740
Rationale: Transurethral resection of the prostate or prostate biopsy is the second
most common cause of granulomatous prostatitis. The disorder results from systemic
granulomatous diseases in fewer than five percent of cases. For these reasons and
because the patient is asymptomatic observation is the most appropriate management.

34
Male Infertility

Randall B. Meacham, Larry I. Lipschultz, Stuart S. Howards

1. **A history of which surgical procedure would *not* commonly be associated with decreased male fertility is:**

    a. bladder neck, Y-V-plasty.
    b. unilateral orchiopexy.
    c. retroperitoneal lymph node dissection.
    d. ureteral reimplantation.
    e. transurethral resection of the prostate.

    Correct Answer: d   Reference Page: 1759
    Rationale: All of the above surgical procedures except ureteral reimplantation have been associated with decreased male fertility. The surgeries and corresponding defects are as follows:
    bladder neck Y-V-plasty: retrograde ejaculation
    orchiopexy: decreased sperm production
    retroperitoneal lymph node dissection: ejaculatory failure
    transurethral resection of the prostate: retrograde ejaculation

2. **Which of the following hormone profiles is consistent with an isolated germinal cell abnormality?**

    a. Decreased testosterone, decreased LH, normal FSH
    b. Normal testosterone, normal LH, elevated FSH
    c. Decreased testosterone, decreased LH, decreased FSH
    d. Normal testosterone, elevated LH, normal FSH
    e. Normal testosterone, normal LH, decreased FSH

    Correct Answer: b   Reference Page: 1761
    Rationale: Significant, intrinsic abnormalities of the seminal epithelium are often reflected by an increase in serum FSH. This elevation of serum FSH is thought to be due to decreased production of inhibin and increased production of activin by the Sertoli cells of the testis. An elevated FSH is a poor prognostic sign in male infertility patients.

3. **Which of the following statements pertaining to varicoceles is *not* correct?**

   a. Varicoceles occur in 15% to 20% of normal males.
   b. Approximately 40% of subfertile men have varicoceles.
   c. All clinically identifiable varicoceles should be repaired.
   d. The left internal spermatic vein is 8 to 10 cm longer than the right.
   e. Varicocele repair is associated with improved semen quality in some patients.

Correct Answer: c   Reference Pages: 1761 and 1778

Rationale: Varicocele repair has been associated with improvement in semen quality in a significant proportion of men and is more common in the subfertile population than the general population. Still, some men with varicocele do not appear to suffer from decreased fertility and thus probably do not require varicocele correction. Relative indications for varicocele repair include decreased semen quality, testicular atrophy, and testicular pain.

4. **The following semen analysis was obtained in a male patient. Which value would *not* be considered abnormal?**

   a. Volume = 1.75 ml
   b. Concentration = 16 x 10^6/ml
   c. Motility = 65%
   d. Forward progression = 1+
   e. Morphology – 45%

Correct Answer: c   Reference Page: 1762

Rationale: This patient was found to have normal mortility but all other values were below the normal range. A properly performed semen analysis obtained on two separate occasions is critical to the male fertility evaluation.

5. **Which of the following is an appropriate use for testis biopsy in the fertility patient?**

   a. To select pharmacologic therapy in the oligospermic patient
   b. To determine the cause of hypospermatogenesis
   c. To establish the prognosis prior to vasectomy reversal
   d. To identify the azoospermic patient that may benefit from surgical therapy
   e. To confirm a diagnosis of hypogonadotropic hypogonadism

Correct Answer: d   Reference Page: 1767

Rationale: With few exceptions, the role of testis biopsy in evaluation of the infertile male is to determine the status of spermatogenesis in the azoospermic patient. If spermatogenesis is found to be intact, the patient may be a candidate for microsurgical reconstruction.

6.   A patient presents with normal physical examination, normal gonadotropins, decreased ejaculate volume, and severe oligoasthenospermia. Evaluation of post-ejaculate urine is negative for sperm. The next step in evaluation should be:

a. MRI of the sella turcica
b. Scrotal ultrasound to rule out varicocele
c. Transrectal ultrasound of the prostatic region and seminal vesicals
d. Bilateral testis biopsy
e. Hamster egg penetration assay to evaluate sperm function

Correct Answer: c   Reference Page: 1771

Rationale: Patients with ejaculatory duct obstruction often present with decreased ejaculate volume and oligoasthenospermia or azoospermia. Transrectal sonography is a readily available, non-invasive method for identifying patients with this lesion. Transurethral resection of the ejaculatory ducts can yield marked improvement in semen quality in this patient population.

7.   **Which of the following fertility related conditions indicates a need for detailed genetic evaluation prior to definitive therapy?**

a. Kallman's syndrome
b. Immunologic infertility (presence of antisperm antibodies)
c. Cryptorchidism
d. Vasal agenesis
e. Ejaculatory duct obstruction

Correct Answer: d   Reference Page: 1783

Rationale: More than 50% of patients found to have congenital bilateral absence of the vas deferens (CBAVD) will be found to have cystic fibrosis trait on DNA evaluation. The carrier rate for this trait in the general population is 1 in 25. Men with CBAVD should be tested for CF trait. Those who are positive should be made aware of this and their partners tested for CF trait before proceeding with sperm aspiration and in vitro fertilization.

35
Strictures of the Male Urethra
Stuart S. Howards

1. **The blood supply of the male urethra is from the:**

a. dorsal artery of the penis, a branch of the internal pudendal artery.
b. bulbar artery, a branch of the inferior vesical artery.
c. dorsal artery of the penis, a branch of the internal pudendal artery and the bulbar artery, a branch of the inferior vesical artery.
d. dorsal artery of the penis, a branch of the internal pudendal artery and the bulbar artery, a branch of the internal pudendal artery.
e. dorsal artery of the penis, a branch of the inferior vesical artery and the bulbar artery, a branch of the internal pudendal artery.

Correct Answer: d   Reference Page: 1803

Rationale: Both the dorsal artery of the penis and the bulbar artery are branches of the internal pudendal artery, which in turn is a branch of the internal iliac. They both supply the urethra. Although the bulbar artery supplies the bulk of the urethra and the proximal portion, distally the urethra is supplied by the dorsal artery of the penis. The dual supply allows the urethra to be detached at either end without compromising its viability. This dual blood supply is important in urethroplasty.

2. **The frequency of urethral injury in men with a pelvic fracture is:**

a. 5%.
b. 10%.
c. 20%.
d. 35%.
e. 50%.

Correct Answer: b   Reference Page: 1807

Rationale: Although the incidence of complications is generally not clinically critical, it is certainly important that a urologist realize, on the one hand, urethral injuries do occur in a significant fraction of patients with pelvic fractures, and, on the other hand, the majority of such patients do not have a urethral injury. These injuries can vary from urethral contusions to total disruption. It is estimated that approximately 34% of such patients have a partial tear of the urethra.

3.   A 40-year-old man is seen in the emergency room following a motor vehicle accident. He has a pelvic fracture and blood is seen at his urethral meatus. He has an obliterative urethral injury. Before surgical repair, he should have several tests. The most important is a:

a.   sonogram.
b.   cystoscopy.
c.   retrograde urethrogram.
d.   voiding cystogram.
e.   combined retrograde urethrogram and voiding cystogram.

Correct Answer: e   Reference Page: 1808

Rationale: All of these tests might be useful in such a patient. However, before surgery one has to define the obliterative lesion by delineating the normal urethra both proximal and distal to the lesion. This is important in order to plan the surgery. The technique for doing this is discussed in the chapter on pp. 1808 and 1809.

4.   The lengths of a bulbar urethral stricture and a pelvic fracture distraction defect that can be repaired by a direct anastomosis are:

a.   3 cm and 2 cm, respectively.
b.   1 cm and 2 cm, respectively.
c.   1 cm and any length, respectively.
d.   3 cm and 1 cm, respectively.
e.   3 cm and any length, respectively.

Correct Answer: c   Reference Page: 1810

Rationale: In the penile and bulbar urethra, strictures larger than 1 cm should not be repaired by direct anastomosis because one has to create a 2 cm defect in order to have 1 cm of spatulation. A 2 cm defect results in urethral shortening due to the required urethral mobilization. On the contrary, injuries after pelvic fracture dislocation can be fixed regardless of length by direct anastomosis because extensive dissection is definitely required and a number of devices which are described later in this chapter can be used to minimize the penile shortening.

5.   **A 20-year-old man presents with difficulty voiding and a decreased urinary stream. He had a straddle injury 8 years previously. A retrograde urethrogram reveals a 1 cm stricture in the penile urethra. He should have a(n):**

    a.   urethral dilatation.
    b.   optical urethrotomy.
    c.   end-to-end open surgical repair.
    d.   split thickness graft repair.
    e.   flap graft repair.

Correct Answer: a   Reference Page:

Rationale: This gentleman has never had any previous instrumentation or attempted repair. A urethral dilatation is simple and cost effective and certainly should be tried initially. If he requires frequent dilatations, then an optical urethrotomy or a surgical repair would be indicated. Since the stricture is short enough, an end-to-end repair would probably be the best choice for an open approach. If the stricture were longer, then a flap graft repair would be indicated.

6.   **A 48-year-old man presents with a symptomatic 2.5 cm bulbar stricture which has been dilated several times and has been treated three times in the preceding 18 months by optical urethrotomy. The stricture is confirmed with a retrograde urethrogram. The next step in management should be:**

    a.   repeat visual urethrotomy.
    b.   an end-to-end anastomosis.
    c.   a split thickness skin graft tube repair.
    d.   a full thickness skin graft tube repair.
    e.   an island pedicle onlay repair.

Correct Answer: e   Reference Page: 1819

Rationale: This patient should have an onlay island pedicle graft repair. He has failed multiple dilatations and urethrotomies, and it is time to give him a definitive repair. As pointed out in previous questions, a 2.5 cm lesion in the bulbous urethra is too long to repair by end-to-end anastomosis. Split thickness grafts tend to shrink and are not reliable. A full thickness tube repair might work well. However, if it fails, one is left with an obliterated urethra. Therefore, the best option is a vascularized onlay pedicle leaving the roof of the urethra. This has the highest success rate.

7.   **A 28-year-old man presents 6 months after a urethral disruption secondary to a motorcycle accident. He has a large defect. The steps which can be utilized to create a tension-free anastomosis include:**

    a.   circumferential mobilization to the suspensory ligament and separation of the corporeal bodies.

    b.   circumferential mobilization to the suspensory ligament and rerouting the urethra around the corporeal bodies.

    c.   circumferential mobilization to the suspensory ligament and an inferior pubectomy.

    d.   rerouting the urethra around the corporeal bodies and an inferior pubectomy.

    e.   circumferential mobilization to the suspensory ligament, separation of the corporeal bodies or rerouting the urethra around the corporeal bodies and an inferior pubectomy.

Correct Answer: e   Reference Page: 1829

Rationale: Repair of these injuries sometimes is quite straightforward. However, not infrequently it is rather complicated and requires knowing many tricks of the trade. Although in most cases it will not be necessary to use all of the listed manipulations, in the most difficult cases one may have to mobilize the urethra, do an inferior pubectomy and separate the corporeal bodies or reroute the urethra around the corporeal bodies.

36

Urethral Carcinoma

David L. McCullough and Raymond E. Poore

1. **Primary transitional cell carcinoma of the prostate is most readily diagnosed by:**

   a. irritative symptoms of frequency, urgency, and dysuria.
   b. nodularity and induration of the prostate on digital rectal examination.
   c. measurement of prostate specific antigen.
   d. biopsy of the prostatic urethra.
   e. finding hypoechoic regions within the prostate using transrectal ultrasound imaging.

   Correct Answer: d   Reference Page: 1839
   Rationale: Irritative voiding symptoms are associated with a host of urologic pathologies and are quite nonspecific. Digital rectal examination will not detect transitional cell carcinoma of the prostate confined to the urethra. PSA is not elevated in cases of transitional cell carcinoma of the prostate. If a lesion is confined to the prostatic urethra it will not be detected on transrectal ultrasound.

2. **Carcinoma of the anterior urethra in the male:**

   a. constitutes the majority of male urethral carcinomas.
   b. typically presents with distant metastases.
   c. requires partial penectomy.
   d. does not usually recur.
   e. has a cure rate that is dependent on local control.

   Correct Answer: e   Reference Page: 1841
   Rationale: Carcinoma of the anterior urethra constitutes slightly less than 40% of all male urethral carcinomas and uncommonly presents with distant metastases. Treatment options for low stage lesions include transurethral resection, open resection of the involved segment, and laser ablation. More invasive tumors usually require partial penectomy with a 2 cm tumor-free margin. After definitive local treatment, recurrence is uncommon.

3. **Which of the following statements is true regarding anterior urethral carcinoma in the male?**

   a. 5-year survival is dismal.
   b. Complications of radiation therapy include penile edema, atrophy, and urethral stricture.
   c. Radiation therapy is a frequently utilized treatment modality.

d.   Failure to cure the disease is probably related to the locally invasive nature of the lesion.

e.   Prophylactic inguinal node dissection is standard practice.

Correct Answer: b   Reference Page: 1841-1842

Rationale: The most common problems associated with radiation therapy for anterior urethral carcinoma include penile edema, penile atrophy, and urethral stricture. Five-year survival is 50%. Radiotherapy is uncommonly used secondary to the high five year survival rate with surgical therapy. Failure to cure is thought to be related to undetected nodal spread at the time of initial surgery. Historically, morbidity from inguinal node dissection has resulted in its use only in the presence of adenopathy or positive biopsy. Reevaluation of indications for prophylactic node dissection is currently in progress.

4.   **Urethral recurrence after cystectomy in patients with transitional cell carcinoma of the bladder is most common in patients whose specimens demonstrated:**

a.   multifocal tumors.
b.   tumors at the bladder neck.
c.   carcinoma in situ.
d.   tumors in the prostate.
e.   tumors at the urethral orifice.

Correct Answer: d   Reference Page: 1845

Rationale: Recent studies have documented urethral recurrence in up to 37% of patients with tumors in the prostate. None of the other choices have recurrence rates approaching this number.

5.   **Primary malignant melanoma of the male urethra is notable for all of the following *except*:**

a.   tumors tend to occur in younger individuals.
b.   tumors are most common in the fossa navicularis.
c.   dissemination is common by direct extension, lymphatics, or hematogenous routes.
d.   survival is poor.
e.   the most beneficial therapy is unknown.

Correct Answer: a   Reference Page: 1845

Rationale: Tumors tend to occur in individuals in their sixties or eighties. The remaining choices are true.

6.   **Which of the following is *not* true about female urethral carcinoma?**

a. Preoperative radiation therapy confers a survival advantage.
b. Bladder preservation may be possible in patients with Stage B or locally advanced C disease.
c. Prophylactic node dissection provides no survival advantage.
d. Treatment prognoses depend on location, size, and stage.
e. Preliminary evidence indicates that chemotherapy may have demonstrable action.

Correct Answer: a　　　　Reference Page: 1849

Rationale: As is common with this uncommon disease, numbers in series are small and studies conflict, but preoperative radiation therapy has not been conclusively shown to provide a survival advantage. Bladder preservation may be possible in patients with Stage B and C disease, even of the entire urethra, as long as the bladder itself is not involved. The remaining choices are true.

7. **When managing the retained urethra of a patient who has undergone cystectomy for transitional cell carcinoma of the bladder, all of the following are true *except*:**

a. a bloody urethral discharge is the most common symptom of urethral recurrence
b. when performing urethrectomy, the fossa navicularis can be left intact for cosmesis.
c. urethral washings must be performed every six months.
d. urethroscopy and urethrograms have a low degree of accuracy in detecting recurrence.
e. the best method of surveillance in patients with continent diversion via an intact urethra is unknown.

Correct Answer: b　　　　Reference Page: 1844-1845

Rationale: The fossa navicularis must always be removed when performing urethrectomy. In one study, 26% of patients who previously underwent urethrectomy were found to have recurrence at the meatal remnant.

37
Gynecological Aspects of Urology

Edward J. McGuire, Marko Gudziak,
Helen O'Connell, Vaseem Ali

1. **In the upright position the normal axis of the upper one third of the vagina is:**

    a. virtually horizontal.
    b. 90° to the horizontal.
    c gently curved posteriorly.
    d. 45° to the horizontal.
    e. slightly anterior to the horizontal.

    Correct Answer: a   Reference Page: 1853
    Rationale: Normally, the upper one third of the vagina is nearly horizontal in the standing position. The upper vagina and rectum usually rest on the levator plate. In genital prolapse, the upper vagina may become vertical and herniate through the potential space in the levator ani muscle. Therefore only A is correct.

2. **A 59-year-old woman develops incontinence after repair of a grade 3 dumbbell shaped cystocele. This is most likely due to:**

    a. motor urge incontinence.
    b. partial bladder denervation associated with the cystocele repair.
    c. exposure of a weak urethra by cystocele repair.
    d. stress incontinence related to urethral denervation.
    e. overflow incontinence.

    Correct Answer: c   Reference Page: 1854
    Rationale: The most common cause of the onset of urinary incontinence after repair of a large cystocele is underlying urethral dysfunction which is unmasked by definitive reduction of the cystocele unless the urethral disorder is also treated. Cystocele repair should not cause incontinence due to urethral and bladder innervation. Cystocele repair is typically associated with improvement in both bladder emptying and motor urge incontinence. Thus a weak urethra with either urethral hypermobility or intrinsic sphincter deficiency is likely to be the cause in this setting.

3.   A **41-year-old woman presents with intermittent severe right sided flank and abdominal pain 22 months following a hysterectomy and bilateral salpingo-oophorectomy done for extensive endometriosis. An IVP shows a dilated right ureter extending into the true pelvis. The next step in diagnosis would be:**

    a.   a serum estradiol and gonadotrophin level of estrogen replacement therapy.
    b.   an antegrade nephrostogram.
    c.   a CT scan.
    d.   laparoscopy.
    e.   an exploratory laparotomy.

Correct Answer: a   Reference Page: 1867

Rationale: The diagnosis to be excluded is ongoing endometriosis causing right ureteral obstruction. After bilateral salpingo–oophorectomy there should be no remaining ovarian tissue. If, however, a retained ovarian fragment exists, hormonal production may continue thereby activating endometrial implants. A serum estradiol and gonadotrophin level after withdrawal of hormone replacement indicate whether castration has been complete. A nephrostogram is unlikely to add to the information gained at IVP and a CT cannot usually detect a retained fragment. Neither laparoscopy nor laparotomy should be used until the diagnosis is clarified.

4.   A **31-year-old woman complains of severe bladder urgency and frequency without incontinence, which is cyclic in nature, occurring just prior to the onset of her menses. The next step in diagnosis would be:**

    a.   urine culture for acid fast organisms.
    b.   cystoscopy and bladder hydrodistention.
    c.   a urinary cytology.
    d.   cell mediated immunologic system testing.
    e.   cystoscopy and laparoscopy together.

Correct Answer: e   Reference Page: 1864-1865

Rationale: The cyclical nature of the irritative bladder symptoms makes endometriosis affecting the bladder the most probable diagnosis. Although the same symptoms without a cyclic pattern indicate interstitial cystitis laparoscopy and cystoscopy will permit a definitive diagnosis to be made and treatment commenced. Genitourinary tuberculosis, HIV infection or other immune suppressive disorders and bladder tumors are all unlikely to cause cyclical symptoms.

5. **A 36-year-old woman presents with right flank pain and has endometriosis demonstrated by laparoscopy which definitely involves the ureter. Treatment of this ureteral obstruction requires:**

a. surgical castration.
b. total abdominal hysterectomy.
c. therapy with GN–RH agonists.
d. estrogen and progestin.
e. surgical resection of the involved ureter and reimplantation.

Correct Answer: e   Reference Page: 1867

Rationale: When ureteral obstruction is due to endometrial involvement of the ureter, definitive treatment of the obstruction with resection of the affected ureteral segment and reimplantation is the only way of preventing a recurrence of the obstruction. Combined hormone therapy, surgical or medical castration may be associated with temporary relief of obstruction but with hormone replacement therapy or with a retained fragment, ureteral disease may recur. A hysterectomy does not treat the ureteral disease.

6. **A 70-year-old woman develops a vesicovaginal fistula 20 years after cessation of radiation therapy for carcinoma of the cervix. The best method of repair would be a(n):**

a. ileal loop diversion.
b. transvesical closure.
c. transperitoneal bladder bivalving procedure.
d. omental interposition.
e. transvaginal approach with a Martius labial fat pad interposition.

Correct Answer: e   Reference Page: 1873

Rationale: A transvaginal approach using a vascularized interposition of labial fat pad would be the least invasive procedure and is associated with excellent results. All other options involve abdominal surgery which in an irradiated patient should be avoided. An ileal loop is a poor solution to this problem associated in the long term with high rate of complications.

7.   A 38-year-old woman complains of incontinence and difficulty voiding 12 months after a radical hysterectomy for cervical carcinoma. An upright cystogram shows a moderate post–voiding residual volume and an open proximal urethra. Management would be best by:

a.   intermittent catheterization.
b.   a needle suspension.
c.   an artificial sphincter.
d.   collagen injection therapy.
e.   a sling and intermittent catheterization.

Correct Answer: e   Reference Page: 1872

Rationale: Radical pelvic surgery may cause bladder decentralization resulting in poor proximal urethral function, detrusor areflexia and poor compliance. Intermittent catheterization alone will not treat poor urethral closure; an artificial sphincter in this setting is prone to causing upper tract deterioration and regardless of which therapy is used to treat the urethral dysfunction, intermittent catheterization is required for bladder emptying. A needle suspension treats urethral hypermobility but does not treat poor proximal urethral closure.

38
Sexually Transmitted Diseases
John N. Krieger

1. **A 19-year-old man complains of dysuria. He is sexually active and had a new partner 7 days ago. Physical exam demonstrates a purulent urethral discharge. A Gram stain of his urethral specimen shows Gram-negative intracellular diplococci. After obtaining specimens for *N. gonorrhoeae* and *C. trachomatis*, the optimal treatment approach is:**

    a. Ceftriaxone 125 mg IM, in a single dose.
    b. Tetracycline, 500 mg, QID for 7 days.
    c. Ciprofloxacin, 500 mg, P.O. in a single dose.
    d. Specitinomycin, 2 g IM, in a single dose.
    e. Cefixime, 400 mg, P.O. in a single dose plus doxycycline, 100 mg, P.O. 2 times a day for seven days.

    Correct Answer: e   Reference Page: 1884
    Rationale: This diagnosis is gonorrhea based on the physical finding of purulent urethral discharge and the Gram stain.

2. **What proportion of men develop gonorrhea following a single episode of vaginal intercourse with an infected woman?**

    a. 0 to 5%
    b. 15% to 20%
    c. 30% to 40%
    d. 50% to 60%
    e. 80% to 90%

    Correct Answer: b   Reference Page: 1882
    Rationale: Approximately 17% of men develop gonorrhea after a single episode of vaginal intercourse with an infected woman. The rate of transmission increases to 60% to 80% after four exposures.

3. **A 21-year-old college student complains of urethral discharge. He is sexually active and had a new sex partner 7 days ago. Physical examination reveals scant, clear urethral discharge. This patient is on spring break vacation and plans to leave the state tomorrow to return to college. You obtain urethral specimens for gonorrhea and chlamydia. The Gram stain reveals multiple polymorphonuclear leukocytes but no intracellular diplococci. The optimal treatment approach is:**

a. Ceftriaxone 125 mg IM, in a single dose.
b. Azithromycin, 500 mg, QID for 7 days.
c. Ciprofloxacin, 500 mg, PO in a single dose.
d. Spectinomycin, 2 g IM, in a single dose.
e. P.O. doxycycline 100 mg, P.O. 2 times a day for seven days.

Correct Answer: e   Reference Page: 1885

Rationale: College students had the lowest reported prevalence (8%) of gonorrhea disease among heterosexual men with urethritis. The presence of scant discharge associated with polymorphonuclear leukocytes but no intracellular diplococci is also consistent with a diagnosis of nongonococcal urethritis. Chlamydia trachomatis is the major differential consideration.

4. **Recommended treatments for acute, nongonococcal urethritis include all of the following *except*:**

a. Doxycycline, 100 mg, orally 2 times a day for 7 days.
b. Azithromycin, 1 g, orally in a single dose.
c. Ofloxacin, 300 mg, orally 2 times a day for 7 days.
d. Ciprofloxacin, 500 mg, orally 2 times a day for 7 days.
e. Erythromycin, 500 mg, orally 4 times a day for 7 days.

Correct Answer: d   Reference Page: 1890

Rationale: Empirical treatment for acute nongonococcal urethritis should be directed primarily against chlamydia trachomatis.

5. **You are treating a 30-year-old man for chlamydial urethritis. He has a 28-year-old wife who is 6 months pregnant. You treat the patient's wife with:**

a. Doxycycline, 100 mg, orally 2 times a day for 7 days.
b. Azithromycin, 1 g, orally in a single dose.
c. Sulfisoxazole, 500 mg, orally 4 times a day for 10 days.
d. Ciprofloxacin, 500 mg, orally 2 times a day for 7 days.
e. Erythromycin, 500 mg, orally 4 times a day for 7 days.

Correct Answer: e   Reference Page: 1890-1891

Rationale: Evaluation of men with chlamydia urethritis should include evaluation and appropriate treatment of sex partners. Because the patient's wife is pregnant, erythromycin is the treatment of choice.

6. **A 35-year-old sexually active woman has painful lesions with a classical appearance for genital herpes. Indications for treatment with oral acyclovir include all of the following *except*:**

a. initial episode of infection.
b. prevention of asymptomatic viral shedding.
c. recurrent episodes in patients with severe symptoms.
d. suppression of recurrent exacerbations in a patient with frequent episodes.
e. a and c

Correct Answer: b   Reference Page: 1897

Rationale: A, C, and D are accepted indications for treatment. Prevention of asymptomatic shedding is not an indicator for treatment.

39
Scrotum and Testis
Randall G. Rowland, Richard S. Foster, John P. Donohue

1. **Hydroceles in adults are frequently tense enough to make examination of their contents difficult or impossible. What is the best way to evaluate the testicle and epididymis inside a tense hydrocele?**

    a.   Manual compression
    b.   Transillumination
    c.   Doppler flow studies
    d.   Scrotal ultrasound scan
    e.   DPTA scan

    Correct Answer: d   Reference Page: 1917-1918
    Rationale: Scrotal ultrasound scans confirm the simple fluid nature of a hydrocele while allowing good imaging of the testis and epididymis. Masses within the testis or epididymis can be delineated clearly which helps determine the etiology (or rule out significant pathologic entities as etiologic factors).

2. **Which of the following choices is *false* about the incidence of testicular tumors?**

    a.   The incidence of testis tumors is equal in all racial populations.
    b.   On average, patients with seminoma present later than those with embryonal carcinoma.
    c.   The right testis is involved more frequently than the left.
    d.   Seminomas have a higher incidence in rural vs. urban areas.
    e.   The incidence of testis cancer is rising with time.

    Correct Answer: a   Reference Page: 1919-1920
    Rationale: Many studies have shown that there is a 2-3 fold difference in the incidence of testicular tumors among racial populations with white populations having the highest incidence.

3. **What is the most common symptom or finding with testicular tumors at the time of diagnosis?**

    a.   Testicular pain
    b.   Scrotal swelling
    c.   Sensation of heaviness of the scrotum
    d.   Hematocele
    e.   Bilateral gynecomastia

Correct Answer: b   Reference Page: 1924
Rationale: Although all of these symptoms and findings can be present at the time the diagnosis is made, scrotal swelling is present most frequently.

4. **If during a transcrotal procedure a testicular tumor is suspected and subsequently confirmed after orchiectomy, what action should be taken if the patient is a clinical stage I and a RPLND is planned for surgical staging?**

    a.   Neoadjuvant chemotherapy should be given.
    b.   The cord structures should be removed through an inguinal incision.
    c.   A hemiscrotectomy should be done.
    d.   A superficial inguinal node dissection should be done.
    e.   Both a hemiscrotectomy and superficial inguinal LND should be done.

Correct Answer: c   Reference Page: 1926
Rationale: Unless there is gross tumor spillage, superficial inguinal nodal involvement is rare. Therefore, removal of the hemiscrotum in addition to the removal of the cord structures which is routinely part of the RPLND is sufficient.

5. **With the use of serum markers (AFP and B-HCG), chest x-rays, tomograms, or CT scans, and abdominal-pelvic CT scans, which answer best describes the incidence and circumstances of understaging?**

    a.   10% of patients who are observed only will relapse.
    b.   30% of patients will have positive nodes at RPLND.
    c.   30% who have negative nodes at RPLND will have a chest relapse.
    d.   50% of patients with testis tumors have negative markers.
    e.   30% of metastases don't show on CT scans due to a 2 cm limit of resolution.

Correct Answer: b   Reference Page: 1928, 1932
Rationale: Of all patients that are clinical stage I, 30% have positive nodes in the retroperitoneum at RPLND. This also correlates with about a 30% failure rate in observation series.

6. **Modification of the RPLND to a prospective nerve sparing technique has increased the incidence of preservation of intact sexual function by preservation of which structures?**

    a.   Lumbar sympathetic chains
    b.   Postganglionic lumbar sympathetic fibers
    c.   Plexus around the origin of the inferior mesenteric artery
    d.   Sympathetic nerves crossing the aortic bifurcation
    e.   All portions of the lumbar and pelvic sympathetic nerves

Correct Answer: e   Reference Page: 1931-1932
Rationale: The RPLND has evolved through modified template techniques which spared one sympathetic chain and its postganglionic fibers to prospective nerve sparing techniques which can be applied to modified or full templates. Sexual function is intact in >98% using this new technique.

7.   **Patients with advanced (stage III) or bulky (stage IIC) testis cancer get the most favorable outcome when treated by which of the following sequences? R.O. - radical orchiectomy; S.C. = systemic chemotherapy; P.C. = post chemotherapy; CR = complete response; PR = partial response**

a.   R.O., S.C., if CR then observation or if PR then PC-RPLND
b.   R.O., RPLND + thoracotomy
c.   S.C., PC-RPLND
d.   R.O., RPLND, S.C.
e.   R.O., RPLND + thoracotomy, S.C.

Correct Answer: a   Reference Page: 1936-1940
Rationale: Experience in many centers has shown that primary chemotherapy followed by surgery if a C.R. is not achieved offers the best overall results. An orchiectomy to remove the primary tumor is needed to avoid possible re-seeding from a sheltered site.

40

The Penis: Sexual Function and Dysfunction

George S. Benson and Michel A. Boileau

1. **Cyclic guanosine monophosphate (GMP) mediated relaxation of penile corporal smooth muscle is stimulated by:**

   a. norepinephrine.
   b. dopamine.
   c. serotonin.
   d. nitric oxide.
   e. endothelin.

   Correct Answer: d   Reference Page: 1959

   Rationale: Relaxation of penile corporal smooth muscle is thought to be a nonadrenergic, noncholinergic mediated event. Recently, the importance of endothelium derived relaxation factor (EDRF) has been recognized. This endothelium dependent relaxation is mediated by nitric oxide. The relaxation produced by nitric oxide is associated with increased intracellular levels of cyclic guanosine monophosphate (GMP). Relaxant responses to nitric oxide are enhanced by pretreating the smooth muscle strips with a cyclic GMP phosphodiesterase inhibitor. Nitric oxide synthase, the enzyme that catalyzes nitric oxide production, has been identified in the pelvic plexus, cavernous nerves and their terminal endings within the corporal erectile tissue, branches of the dorsal penile nerves, and nerve plexuses in the adventitia of the deep cavernosal arteries in man. Nitric oxide, therefore, does appear to be an important mediator of corporal smooth muscle relaxation. Norepinephrine and endothelin cause contraction of corporal smooth muscle.

2. **Hypogonadal men receiving parenteral testosterone should be monitored by periodic measurement of PSA, liver function tests, and:**

   a. white blood cell count.
   b. bleeding time.
   c. prothrombin time.
   d. hematocrit.
   e. platelet count.

   Correct Answer: d   Reference Page: 1970

   Rationale: Patients receiving long-term intramuscular testosterone therapy should be monitored for the development of complications from this therapy. Parenteral testosterone is contraindicated in the presence of prostate cancer, and patients receiving testosterone should be monitored with digital rectal examination and serum prostate specific antigen determination. Although hepatotoxicity has been markedly reduced when esterified rather than alkylated testosterone is used, evaluation of liver function studies before and periodically during therapy is prudent. Androgen therapy has also been demonstrated to increase hematocrit and red blood cell volume by stimulating erythropoietin production. Patients with hematocrit values greater than 48% do appear to be at risk for cardiovascular complications. The patient's hematocrit should therefore be monitored. Testosterone does not appear to have a significant effect on the white blood cell count, bleeding time, prothrombin time, or platelet count.

3.   **Neurologic testing with sacral evoked potentials evaluates:**

   a.   parasympathetic afferents and somatic efferents.
   b.   somatic afferents and parasympathetic efferents.
   c.   parasympathetic afferents and sympathetic efferents.
   d.   somatic afferents and somatic efferents.
   e.   sympathetic afferents and parasympathetic efferents.

Correct Answer: d   Reference Page: 1973
Rationale: The sacral evoked potential (sacral latency) is essentially an electrophysio-logic test that measures the bulbocavernosus reflex. In the performance of this test, penile skin is stimulated and recordings are made from a needle electrode placed in the bulbocavernosus muscle. The afferent limb of this reflex is therefore somatic sensory and the efferent limb is somatic efferent. Penile erection is governed by a reflex arc consisting of pudendal afferent (sensory) fibers and parasympathetic efferent (motor) fibers. The sensory portion of the reflex that governs erection and the sensory portion of the reflex which is measured by sacral evoked potentials are therefore identical. The efferent (parasympathetic) portion of the reflex controlling erection cannot be accurately evaluated by currently available studies. The sacral evoked response therefore measures reflex activity over the pudendal (somatic) sensory nerves and the pudendal (somatic) motor nerves. This study provides information concerning some reflex activity through the sacral spinal cord, but it does not directly assess efferent penile innervation.

4.   **A 55-year-old man is participating in a self intracavernosal injection program for impotence. He is hypertensive and 4 years ago he suffered a myocardial infarction. After the intracorporal injection of 10 mcg of PGE$_1$, he develops priapism. The safest drug to inject intracorporally to treat his priapism is:**

   a.   phenylephrine.
   b.   epinephrine.
   c.   norepinephrine.
   d.   metaraminol.
   e.   ephedrine.

Correct Answer: a   Reference Page: 1974

Rationale: Of all the drugs listed, phenylephrine is the purest α-adrenergic agonist. Epinephrine, norepinephrine, and ephedrine have significant β-adrenergic activity and the potential, therefore, for more cardiac toxicity than does phenylephrine. Several deaths have been reported following the intracorporal injection of metaraminol. Phenylephrine appears to be a relatively safe agent, but because of the potential for significant cardiovascular morbidity, all of these agents should be used with care.

5. **A 60-year-old man has a 5-year history of Peyronie's disease. He has a 2 cm x 3 cm stable plaque on the dorsum of his penis and is unable to achieve any degree of penile tumescence. He desires therapy. The best next step is:**

    a.   color Doppler ultrasound.

    b.   cavernosometry and cavernosography.

    c.   plaque excision and dermal graft.

    d.   plaque excision and tunica vaginalis graft.

    e.   placement of penile prosthesis.

Correct Answer: e   Reference Page: 1986

Rationale: In patients with Peyronie's disease and impotence, most authors advocate the placement of a penile prosthesis with or without a penile straightening procedure. The performance of a color Doppler ultrasound or cavernosometry and cavernosography does not really change the approach to therapy in these patients. Plaque excision with either a dermal or a tunica vaginalis graft is usually reserved for those patients with Peyronie's disease, significant penile deformity, and adequate erectile function.

6. **Twelve hours after sustaining blunt perineal trauma, a 20-year-old man develops painless priapism. Corporal aspiration yields bright red blood. The best management of his priapism is:**

    a.   intracavernosal phenylephrine.

    b.   glans penis-cavernosal shunt (Winter).

    c.   saphenous vein-cavernosal shunt (Grayhack).

    d.   cavernospongiosum shunt (Quackels).

    e.   angiographic arterial embolization.

Correct Answer: e   Reference Page: 1984

Rationale: The patient described most likely has high flow priapism. He experienced perineal trauma and has a painless erection. Corporal aspiration yielded bright red blood which is consistent with a high flow state. The diagnosis can be confirmed by color Doppler ultrasound. Patients with high flow priapism are best treated by angiographic arterial embolization of the injured vessel. Although transient detumescence may occur with the intracavernosal instillation of phenylephrine, and the priapism generally recurs. The surgical shunting procedures are reserved for patients with low flow priapism.

7. **A 40-year-old man with end stage renal disease has erectile dysfunction. He is on dialysis, but expects to undergo renal transplantation within the next 6 months. The best next step in management of his impotence is:**

a.   reevaluate after renal transplantation.
b.   placement of an inflatable penile prosthesis.
c.   placement of a semi-rigid penile prosthesis.
d.   color Doppler ultrasound.
e.   cavernosometry and cavernosography.

Correct Answer: a   Reference Page: 1965
Rationale: The incidence of erectile dysfunction in patients with chronic renal failure who are on dialysis is very high. After renal transplantation, most patients do report a return to preillness levels of sexual activity. Improved erectile function has been described in 70% to 80% of patients. The reasons for improvement in sexual function following transplantation are not known, but are hypothesized to be related to increased levels of serum testosterone, vascular and neural effects, or to an improvement in a generalized sense of well being.

8. **Priapism is a well-recognized side effect in patients treated with:**

a.   trazodone.
b.   cimetidine.
c.   propranolol.
d.   reserpine.
e.   methyldopa

Correct Answer: a   Reference Page: 1973
Rationale: Trazodone, an antidepressant agent, is associated with priapism in a significant number of patients. For this reason, this antiserotoninergic drug has been advocated for the treatment of erectile dysfunction. Patients taking trazodone should be warned of this complication and seek urologic help if a persistent erection occurs. The other drugs listed—cimetidine, propranolol, resperine, and methyldopa—are all agents which have been associated with impotence, not priapism.

41
Benign and Malignant Lesions of the Penis
Mark Chazen and Gerald Sufrin

1. **In the treatment of the primary penile lesion of squamous cell cancer of the penis:**

   a. the type of therapy selected, that is radiotherapy vs partial amputation, is an important prognostic factor in ultimate survival.
   b. for lesions invading the corpora, partial amputation with a two cm tumor free margin has the lowest incidence of local recurrence, when compared to other therapies.
   c. local recurrence following organ sparing therapies, e.g., radiotherapy or micrographic surgery, even if detected and treated promptly, is associated with a compromised survival.
   d. bleomycin-based chemotherapy offers a predictably effective option in treating the primary lesion.
   e. brachytherapy as compared to teletherapy offers superior local control and survival.

   Correct Answer: b   Reference Page: 2018
   Rationale: The type of therapy of the primary lesion, assuming adequacy of local control, has not been shown to be an important prognostic factor. Similarly, local recurrence if detected promptly and treated definitively has not been associated with a compromised survival. Systemic chemotherapy using bleomycin has not proven effective in predictably providing local tumor control and when brachytherapy is compared to teletherapy, no therapeutic superiority has been demonstrated.

   In corporal invasion, partial amputation with a tumor free margin has provided the lowest incidence of local recurrence.

2. **The most likely initial sites of lymph node metastases in a patient with squamous cell cancer of the glans penis include all of the following *except*:**

   a. superficial inguinal nodes.
   b. deep inguinal nodes.
   c. external iliac nodes.
   d. internal (hypogastric) nodes.
   e. obturator nodes.

Correct Answer: a   Reference Page: 2010

Rationale: The lymphatics of the glans, frenulum, urethra and corpora spongiosa drain to the deep (i.e., below the fascia lata) inguinal nodes or directly into the external iliac, hypogastric (internal iliac), or obturator nodes. While the superficial inguinal nodes are not primarily the site of drainage of glandular lesions, these nodes may become involved by retrograde filling.

3. **Following definitive treatment of the primary penile lesion of squamous cell carcinoma of the penis, the optimal management of a 61-year-old patient with a 2 cm x 3 cm palpable left inguinal mass is:**

  a.   bilateral inguinal and pelvic lymphadenectomy within 7 days of treatment of the primary penile lesion.
  b.   a course of a broad spectrum antibiotic for 6 weeks followed by re-evaluation of the nodal status.
  c.   biopsy of the inguinal mass within 7 days of treatment of the primary lesion.
  d.   CT scan of the abdomen and chest to detect other possible sites of adenopathy and/or occult pulmonary lesions.
  e.   bilateral sentinel node biopsy within 7 days of treatment of the primary lesion.

Correct Answer: b   Reference Page: 2025

Rationale: Bilateral pelvic and inguinal lymphadenectomy within 7 days of treatment of the primary lesion is associated with an unacceptably high incidence of infectious complications and does not allow sufficient time for resolution of inflammatory nodes.

Nodal biopsy either by aspiration, open biopsy or by sentinel node biopsy within 7 days of treatment of the primary lesion results in a high percent of inflammatory node biopsies, may be associated with increased risk of infectious complications and may fail to detect metastatic lesions.

CT scan of the abdomen would not include the pelvic nodes and metastases to abdominal nodes (i.e., lumbar node) would be unlikely in the absence of pelvic node metastases.

A 6-week course of a broad spectrum antibiotic would effectively address adenopathy due to infectious etiologies and allow re-evaluation. This would be important if the adenopathy resolved and if a plan of close monitoring rather than prophylactic lymphadenectomy was selected. In addition, and if lymphadenectomy was elected, then infectious complications would be minimized.

4. **Factors which most reliably correlate with prognosis in patients with penile carcinoma include all of the following *except*:**

a. presence or absence of pelvic lymph node metastases.
b. interval of time between initial symptoms of the penile lesion and diagnosis.
c. presence or absence of inguinal lymph node metastases.
d. corporal invasion.
e. tumor grade and/or tumor ploidy.

Correct Answer: b   Reference Page: 2033

Rationale: The presence or absence of lymph node metastases, whether inguinal or pelvic, have in multiple studies been shown to be a strong prognostic factor. Patients with either inguinal or pelvic node metastases have a prognosis clearly inferior to that of patients without metastases.

The presence of corporal invasion which facilitates access to vascular dissemination is associated with a poorer prognosis than the absence of such invasion.

Tumor grade and tumor ploidy have been correlated with prognosis particularly when low grade diploid lesions are compared to high grade aneuploid lesions.

Despite the often prolonged interval between the symptomatic appearance of a penile lesion and its definitive treatment (often several months) no predictable or direct correlation between this interval and prognosis can be demonstrated.

5. **Bowenoid papulosis:**

a. is rarely associated with HPV-16.
b. is usually associated with occult visceral malignancies.
c. rarely leads to invasive squamous cell cancer.
d. is usually found in uncircumcised patients.
e. is best treated by partial penile amputation.

Correct Answer: c   Reference Page: 2002

Rationale: Bowenoid papulosis is a form of carcinoma in situ and is often associated with HPV-16. However, and in contrast to Bowen's disease, it is not associated with visceral malignancies. Interestingly, it is found in circumcised males and it is best treated by organ sparing therapies since it does not progress to invasive penile cancer.

6. **Transplantation of the sartorius muscle following ilioinguinal lymphadenectomy reduces the incidence of:**

a. postoperative wound infection.
b. postoperative lymphedema.
c. delayed postoperative hemorrhage from the femoral vessels.
d. flap necrosis.
e. tumor recurrence in the groin.

Correct Answer: c   Reference Page: 2030

Rationale: Sartorius muscle transplantation (i.e., detachment of the origin of the sartorius muscle and its repositioning to cover the femoral vessels by suturing to the inguinal ligament) has no demonstrable influence on the incidence of postoperative wound infection, lymphedema, cutaneous "flap" necrosis or tumor recurrence in the groin.

Sartorius muscle transplantation, however, clearly reduces the incidence of postoperative and often fatal hemorrhage from the femoral vessels.

42
Dermatologic Lesions of the Penis
B. Dale Wilson and Stuart S. Howards

1. **Which of the following are true regarding benign verruciform xanthomas?**

    a.   Serum cholesterol and triglyceride levels are normal.
    b.   They are associated with diabetes mellitus.
    c.   They usually appear on the scrotum.
    d.   Histologically the squamous epithelium reveals hyperkeratosis, acanthosis, and parakeratosis.
    e.   a and d.

    Correct Answer: e   Reference Page: 2044
    Rationale: Although this is a rare lesion, when it does occur, it often appears on the penis. It is benign and, in spite of its name, it is not associated with elevated lipids of diabetes. Histologically, the epithelium reveals hyperkeratosis, acanthosis, and parakeratosis.

2. **Lichen sclerosis et atrophicus:**

    a.   is never associated with malignancy.
    b.   circumcised males have a lower incidence.
    c.   is associated with a higher incidence of squamous cell carcinoma in males compared to females.
    d.   occurs only in men over 50.
    e.   can be treated by surgical excision.

    Correct Answer: b   Reference Page: 2044-2045
    Rationale: Lichen sclerosis et atrophicus is associated with malignancy in a small percentage of children and in about 5% of women. It is less common in circumcised males. It may occur at any age but is more common in men over 50. It can be treated by surgical excision as well as intralesional and sublesional steroids.

3. **Bowenoid papulosis:**

    a.   is characterized histologically by the features of squamous cell carcinoma in situ.
    b.   occurs more frequently in uncircumcised males.
    c.   can be locally aggressive but does not metastasize.
    d.   therapy includes surgical excision, cryosurgery, CO_2 or neodymium YAG laser surgery, interferon, topical 5-fluouracil.
    e.   all of the above.

Correct Answer: e   Reference Page: 2052-2053

Rationale: All of the listed statements are true regarding Bowen's papillomatosis. It is distinguished from Bowen's disease by its early onset, occurrence in uncircumcised males and multiplicity of lesions. Histologically it has a malignant appearance, but it often has a benign course.

4.   **Giant condylomata acuminata:**

a.   histologically appears benign.
b.   human papilloma virus (tPV) Types 16 and 18 reflect a benign trend.
c.   treatment includes conventional or Mohs micrographic surgery.
d.   can be associated with invasive squamous cell carcinoma and metastasis.
e.   all of the above

Correct Answer: e   Reference Page: 2054

Rationale: All of the statements are true for giant condylomata acuminata. It may extend to the glans, prepuce and shaft of the penis, or it may be localized.

43
General Considerations of Congenital Anomalies
Ronald Rabinowitz

1. **A 38-week gestational age 2000 gram boy is 4 hours old. He has tracheo-esophageal fistula and imperforate anus. A VCUG and retrograde urethrogram demonstrate a normal bladder and urethra. On the VCUG, 2 lumbar hemivertebrae are noted. His physical examination demonstrates a deformed right wrist. The external genital examination is normal. The pediatric surgeon is planning to repair the tracheo-esophageal fistula and perform a diverting colostomy. The next step in the urologic management of this boy is:**

   a. intravenous urogram.
   b. ultrasound examination of the urinary tract.
   c. cystoscopy at the time of surgery.
   d. MRI of the lumbosacral spine.
   e. ultrasound examination of the lumbosacral spine.

   Correct Answer: b   Reference Page: 2062, 2069
   Rationale: This baby has multiple congenital abnormalities. As the number of malformations increases, especially those of the gastrointestinal or skeletal system, the risk for urinary tract involvement also increases. Although this boy will be under anesthesia, there is no radiographic evidence of a rectourethral fistula or bladder abnormality. Cystoscopy would add no useful information at this time, and instrumentation may be dangerous because of the small urethral caliber. If cystoscopy were ultimately necessary, it could be done at a later date in conjunction with anal reconstruction. While the entire spine will need to be evaluated, that can be performed electively. An intravenous urogram is unlikely to be helpful at this early age. The constellation of abnormalities seen in this baby is the VATER Association and has a high risk for renal dysplasia. Ultrasonography is an excellent and rapid way to screen for major urologic abnormalities.

2. **A family had a son with Trisomy 18 Syndrome (Edwards Syndrome) who died at age 7 months of cardiopulmonary disease. He also had a horseshoe kidney, hydronephrosis, hypospadias, and bilateral undescended testes. They plan to attempt to have another child and seek advice regarding prenatal diagnosis. The best way to make such a diagnosis is by:**

   a. fetoscopy.
   b. ultrasonography of the fetal kidneys.
   c. biochemical analysis of the amniotic fluid.
   d. ultrasonography of the fetal genitalia.
   e. fetal chromosomal analysis.

Correct Answer: e   Reference Page: 2063

Rationale: When there has been a previous child with a chromosomal abnormality, especially a trisomy, prenatal screening in future pregnancies is indicated. Amniocentesis and chromosomal analysis of the fetal cells is diagnostic. While ultrasonography may diagnose fetal renal and genital anatomic abnormalities, it will not diagnose a chromosomal anomaly. Similarly, fetoscopy can give gross anatomic information, but will not be diagnostic. Biochemical analysis of the amniotic fluid will not make the diagnosis of a chromosomal abnormality.

3. **A family has a child with myelomeningocele and severe hydronephrosis who underwent continent urinary diversion. The family is contemplating another pregnancy and seeks advice regarding the prenatal diagnosis of another child with a neural tube defect. The best way to make such a diagnosis is by:**

    a.   fetal alpha-fetoprotein levels.
    b.   maternal alpha-fetoprotein levels.
    c.   ultrasonography of the fetal kidneys.
    d.   ultrasonography of the fetal spine.
    e.   chromosomal analysis of the amniotic fluid.

Correct Answer: a   Reference Page: 2063

Rationale: Ultrasonography of the fetal kidneys may demonstrate hydronephrosis, which may be associated with, but is not diagnostic of a neural tube defect. Maternal levels of alpha fetoprotein may suggest this condition. The amniotic fluid is diagnostic, but it must be analyzed for alpha fetoprotein, not chromosomes. Ultrasonography of the fetal spine may anatomically demonstrate a neural tube defect, and should be carried out in conjunction with fetal alpha-fetoprotein levels. However, a smaller defect may not be identified and amniocentesis for alpha fetoprotein levels is diagnostic.

4. **A 2-month-old girl has 2 sisters with vesicoureteral reflux. One required surgical correction for high grade reflux with renal parenchymal loss and the other is being followed on long-term antibacterial prophylaxis. This baby is asymptomatic, the physical examination is normal, and the urine culture is sterile. The best way to determine whether this girl has a familial form of vesicoureteral reflux is by:**

    a.   renal ultrasonography.
    b.   intravenous urography.
    c.   isotope cystography.
    d.   chromosomal analysis.
    e.   cystoscopy.

Correct Answer: c   Reference Page: 2063 , 2067
Rationale: With increasing numbers of siblings with vesicoureteral reflux, the risk for reflux increases. However, the mode of inheritance is probably polygenic. Thus, chromosomal analysis won't help. Both renal ultrasonography and intravenous urography will give excellent anatomic renal information, but neither will diagnose reflux. Cystoscopy is not a diagnostic study in this condition. The information required is whether this asymptomatic individual has reflux and the only study listed to make this diagnosis is the isotope cystogram.

5.   **The best way to follow renal status in children with aniridia, hemihypertrophy, Beckwith-Wiedemann syndrome, or myelodysplasia is with periodic:**

   a.   intravenous urography.
   b.   computed tomography.
   c.   ultrasonography.
   d.   magnetic resonance imaging.
   e.   radioisotope imaging.

Correct Answer: c   Reference Page: 2061
Rationale: Children with aniridia, hemihypertrophy, and Beckwith-Wiedemann syndrome are at significantly increased risk for the development of Wilms' tumor. Children with myelodysplasia are at significantly increased risk for the development of hydronephrosis. Thus, all of these children need periodic anatomic uroradiographic investigation, often multiple times within a year. As a screening study, ultrasonography provides efficient and excellent anatomic information with the least invasiveness.

6.   **Bilateral mild fetal hydronephrosis was diagnosed at 20 weeks gestational age. By 28 weeks, the hydronephrosis was moderate bilaterally and ultrasound demonstrated a male phallus. The urinary bladder was distended on each study. The volume of amniotic fluid was normal. The fetal chest was normal. At 32 weeks, the hydronephrosis was a little more severe bilaterally, with no other changes. The ureters were not seen, but the bladder was still distended. The next step in the management of this fetus is:**

   a.   early delivery at 34 weeks.
   b.   amniocentesis for electrolytes.
   c.   suprapubic cystourethrogram.
   d.   repeat ultrasonography at 36 weeks.
   e.   placement of an indwelling catheter shunt.

Correct Answer: d   Reference Page: 2063

Rationale: There are few indications for diverting the fetal urinary tract with a shunt. These include decreased amniotic fluid volume in addition to worsening hydronephrosis. While posterior urethral valves is a possibility, the presence of normal amniotic fluid volume indicates adequate renal function. Thus contrast radiographic investigation can wait until after delivery. Delivery need not be advanced as long as the amniotic fluid volume remains normal. Electrolyte evaluation of the amniotic fluid may be a less sensitive indicator of fetal renal function and has more potential risks as an invasive study. Since the ureters may not be dilated, this boy may have bilateral ureteropelvic junction obstruction. Thus, this fetus may be safely followed until term, then evaluated in the newborn period.

44
Perinatal Urology
Marc Cendron

1.   Urine production by the fetal kidneys:

a.   is regulated by the placenta.
b.   is decreased in the fetus of a diabetic mother.
c.   starts between gestation weeks 9 and 12.
d.   starts between gestation weeks 12 and 16.
e.   is stimulated by renin.

Correct Answer: c   Reference Pages: 2078-2088
Rationale: Urine formation by the fetal kidney begins between 9 and 12 weeks of gestation and has been documented by distention of the renal pelvis (Potter, 1972). The placenta, renin or the presence of maternal diabetes do not appear to affect fetal urine production.

2.   GFR in the fetus:

a.   is determined by the volume of amniotic fluid.
b.   is not dependent on the permeability of the glomerular wall.
c.   quadruples between gestational age 26 and 40 weeks.
d.   remains stable after birth.
e.   is autoregulated.

Correct Answer: c   Reference Pages: 2079-2081
Rationale: Glomerular filtration rate in the fetus increases progressively with gestational age (Smith et. al, 1993). Fetal GFR appears to be dependent on several factors that include the permeability of the glomerular wall, the surface area available for filtration and the ultrafiltration pressure that is dependent on afferent arterial resistance, capillary blood flow, and the protein concentration in arterial plasma (Guignard and John, 1986). Recently, Wilkins (1992), confirmed that GFR quadruples between gestational age 26 and 40 weeks. After birth the GFR continues to mature slowly and progressively for approximately four months after birth.

3.   Fetal renal dysplasia:

a.   is associated with obstructive uropathy occurring late in gestation.
b.   is characterized by organized metanephrine structures.
c.   is present in fetal kidneys with cortical cysts.
d.   is always associated with high grade vesicoureteral reflux.
e.   can be reliably identified on prenatal ultrasound.

Correct Answer: c   Reference Pages: 2098-2099
Rationale: Dysplastic fetal kidneys are characterized by an increased echogenicity on ultrasound but the sonographic detection of cortical cysts implies the presence of severe dysplasia and indicates irreversible renal damage. More than 90% of dysplastic kidneys with cortical cysts are associated with an obstructive process occurring early in nephrogenesis (Ruben-Stein et. al, 1961). Cortical cysts have been shown by Mahoney et. al (1994) to have a higher positive predictive value for renal dysplasia.

4.   **On prenatal ultrasound, the echographic criterion that correlates best with a functionally significant renal lesion is:**

a.   stable hydronephrosis.
b.   renal parenchymal thinning.
c.   increased renal echogenicity.
d.   caliectasis.
e.   ureteral dilatation.

Correct Answer: c   Reference Pages: 2084-2085
Rationale: Fetal renal function can be inferred from three parameters:
1) measurement of fetal urine output, 2) sonographic appearance of the kidney, and 3) analysis of fetal urine composition after percutaneous aspiration. The sonographic detection of cortical cysts and increased cortical echogenicity have been associated with irreversible renal damage in the fetus (Mahoney et. al, 1994). It should be noted that normal fetal kidneys beyond 30 weeks gestation exhibit, on ultrasound, an echo-texture similar to that of the liver with an internal architecture showing a differentiation between cortex and medulla. In contrast, a dysplastic kidney exhibits no internal architecture and may have increased echogenicity caused by disruption in normal histology. More than 90% of dysplastic kidneys with cortical cysts are associated with an obstructive process occurring usually early on in nephrogenesis.

5.   **Fetuses with prenatal dilatation of the urinary tract and poor postnatal renal function produce, in utero:**

a.   isotonic urine.
b.   hypertonic urine.
c.   hypotonic urine.
d.   reduced amounts of beta 2 microglobulins.
e.   excessive amounts of hydrogen ions.

Correct Answer: a   Reference Pages: 2084-2085
Rationale: Fetal urine is an ultrafiltrative fetal serum. Observations by Glick and coworkers (1985) showed that fetuses with congenital hydronephrosis and normal renal function produced hypotonic urine whereas those with poor function made urine that was isotonic. These observations were obtained after a study from the Fetal

Treatment Program in San Francisco in which 20 fetuses with bilateral hydronephrosis
were evaluated, 18 of which had percutaneous drainage of fetal urine prior to birth.

6. **In a newborn with dyspnea and a pneumothorax noted on chest x-ray, the most
    likely urologic diagnosis is:**

    a. a UPJ obstruction with very large renal pelvis.
    b. a large multicystic dysplastic kidney.
    c. small bowel obstruction.
    d. severe urethral obstruction.
    e. VACTERL syndrome.

Correct Answer: d   Reference Page: 2131

Rationale: The newborn with posterior urethral valves may have an abdominal mass,
failure to thrive, urosepsis, or urinary ascites as presenting signs and symptoms. In
addition, dyspnea at birth associated with a pneumothorax or pneumomediastinum may
be the initial sign of severe urethral obstruction (Nakayama et. al, 1986 and Renert
et. al 1972). When the diagnosis of posterior urethral valves is suspected, urethral
catheterization should be performed and a VCUG should be obtained. An ultrasound
of the bladder and kidney is also very important in the evaluation of these patients.

7. **Renal failure should be suspected in a newborn who has:**

    a. a serum creatinine of 1.1 mg/dl 12 hours after birth.
    b. not voided within 24 hours after birth.
    c. not voided within 48 hours after birth.
    d. a sustained decrease in urine output less than 3 ml/kg/hr.
    e. bilateral hydronephrosis on postnatal ultrasound.

Correct Answer: c   Reference Page: 2138

Rationale: Acute renal failure should be suspected in any infant who has a sustained
decrease in urine output less than 1 ml/kg/hr and persistent serum creatinine levels
greater than 1 mg/dl (in newborns beyond 34 weeks gestation), or who has hematuria.
Although renal failure may be associated with normal or even increased production
of urine, most neonates with acute renal failure have oliguria or anuria. As far as
voiding is concerned, 92% of term newborns pass urine within 24 hours of birth, and
99.4% within 48 hours. An infant who has not voided within the first 48 hours of life
should therefore be suspected of having renal failure. In addition, 12 hours after birth,
a serum creatinine of 1.1 is still reflective of mother's creatinine. Bilateral hydronephrosis is rarely associated with renal failure except in cases of severe posterior
urethral valve or UPJ obstruction.

8.   **Neonatal testicular torsion:**

a.   is intravaginal.
b.   is extravaginal.
c.   presents as a painful, soft scrotal mass.
d.   requires immediate exploration.
e.   should be approached through the scrotum.

Correct Answer: b   Reference Page: 2146

Rationale: In most cases, a hard, nontender scrotal mass that is present at birth represents a testicular torsion. Anatomically, testicular torsion in the newborn is extravaginal with twisting of the entire spermatic cord in contrast to pubertal boys in whom testicular torsion is usually intravaginal. It usually presents as a non-painful mass and usually does not require emergent scrotal exploration. It should be approached through an inguinal incision.

45
Anomalies of the Kidney
Stephen A. Koff

1. **With respect to ureteropelvic junction obstruction, which of the following is true?**

    a.   A kidney with a small renal pelvis is at greater risk for subsequent deterioration than a kidney with a very large renal pelvis.

    b.   Fifty percent of neonates with hydronephrosis will ultimately require pyeloplasty.

    c.   Visualization of a normal distal ureter excludes ureteropelvic junction obstruction.

    d.   Nearly all patients demonstrate measurable radiographic improvement in function after pyeloplasty.

    e.   Other coexistent genitourinary pathology is usually present.

Correct Answer: a   Reference Pages: 2185-2186

Rationale: Recent series emphasizing an initial nonoperative approach have shown that the majority of neonates with hydronephrosis will have adequate drainage and maintain function in extended follow-up. The reasons for this are partly explained by experimental studies which have shown that partial obstruction may lead to an increase in size of the renal pelvis as a compensatory mechanism. The dilated collecting system, especially if it is extrarenal, will be highly compliant dampening any diuresis-induced intrapelvic pressure changes and thus preserving function.

2. **Potter's syndrome due to bilateral renal agenesis is usually associated with which of the following?**

    a.   Pulmonary hypoplasia

    b.   Characteristic hand deformity

    c.   Absent adrenal glands

    d.   Absence of the clavicles

    e.   Urinary ascites

Correct Answer: a   Reference Pages: 2171-2172

Rationale: Potter's syndrome refers to a group of findings in neonates with severe oligohydramnios of any etiology. The syndrome is characterized by pulmonary hypoplasia, bowed and clubbed legs, facial deformities and an absent or hypoplastic urinary system. The adrenal glands are typically present. It is felt that the features of the syndrome are due to the mechanical compression on the fetus from a lack of sufficient amniotic fluid.

3. **Renal blood supply is normal in:**

a. pelvic kidney.
b. horseshoe kidney.
c. crossed renal ectopia.
d. thoracic kidney.
e. multicystic dysplastic kidney.

Correct Answer: d   Reference Page: 2177

Rationale: Kidneys in ectopic locations typically have a very anomalous blood supply. This fact must be kept in mind if open renal surgery is contemplated. Kidneys are very rarely located in the thorax but when they are, have normal renal vessels.

4. **One year after onset of normal menarche, a 13-year-old girl develops pelvic pain with menstrual irregularity. An ultrasound demonstrates a pelvic mass and a solitary right kidney. Which of the following is most likely?**

a. Uterine atresia
b. Imperforate hymen with obstruction
c. Uterus didelphys with obstruction
d. Ovarian cyst
e. Appendiceal abscess

Correct Answer: c   Reference Page: 2172

Rationale: In a teenager who initially had normal menses, a pelvic mass with a solitary kidney most likely represents uterus didelphys with obstruction of a hemivagina. In unilateral renal agenesis genital anomalies occur three to four times more commonly in females than males and are usually secondary to partial or complete nonunion of the Mullerian ducts. The other choices listed would either not lead to menstrual irregularities or would not have allowed a period of normal menstruation.

5. **With regard to horseshoe kidneys:**

a. Most cases require surgery.
b. If UPJ obstruction is diagnosed, division of the isthmus is required to ensure adequate dependent drainage.
c. Horseshoe kidneys are commonly associated with other genitourinary pathology.
d. Dysplasia and neoplasia are common.
e. Hydronephrosis usually represents UPJ obstruction.

Correct Answer: c   Reference Pages: 2179-2181

Rationale: Other abnormalities, including genitourinary ones are often found in children with horseshoe kidneys. Due to their bizarre appearance and the high rate of hydronephrosis, early studies suggested that most cases required surgery. Later series have demonstrated that most patients can be followed nonoperatively with surgery reserved for those few who have functional impairment or recurrent infections. The isthmus often contains functioning tissue and division carries some risk and should not be routinely performed during pyeloplasty. Though there is an increased risk of dysplasia and neoplasia, they are not commonly found.

6.   **Abnormalities associated with megacalycosis include:**

    a.   ureterovesical junction obstruction.
    b.   ureteropelvic junction obstruction.
    c.   tubular concentrating defect.
    d.   renal cortical scarring.
    e.   renal dysplasia.

Correct Answer: c   Reference Pages: 2181-2182

Rationale: Patients with megacalycosis have a tubular concentrating defect, an underdeveloped medulla, dilated calyces but a normal renal pelvis with no obstruction at the ureteropelvic or ureterovesical junction.

7.   **In extrinsic ureteropelvic junction obstruction:**

    a.   the obstruction is often associated with aberrant vessels or fibrous bands.
    b.   removal of the extrinsic tissue will lead to resolution of the obstruction.
    c.   upper tract urodynamics suggests a pressure-dependent obstruction.
    d.   obstruction is usually present continuously.
    e.   the ureteropelvic junction is usually anatomically normal.

Correct Answer: a   Reference Pages: 2177-2189

Rationale: In extrinsic obstruction, aberrant bands or vessels result in a kinking of the ureteropelvic junction. However, there is also usually an associated intrinsic narrowing or stenosis that must likewise be corrected. Obstruction is often present intermittently and is related to the volume of the renal pelvis. Sudden diuresis may increase the degree of kinking at the extrinsic fixed point transiently exacerbating the obstruction.

8.   **With regard to renal vascular abnormalities:**

a.   Most renovascular fistulas are secondary to ruptured renal artery aneurysms.

b.   Saccular renal aneurysms in adults usually result from post-stenotic flow disturbances.

c.   An asymptomatic renal arterial aneurysm that is 3.0 cm in size should be surgically repaired.

d.   Post-traumatic arteriovenous fistulae require surgical correction.

e.   Congenital arteriovenous malformations usually present in childhood.

Correct Answer: c   Reference Pages: 2192-2193

Rationale: An asymptomatic renal aneurysm that is either greater than 2.5 cm in size, incompletely calcified or associated with uncontrolled hypertension should be repaired. Saccular aneurysms are the most common forms in adults and are due to a weakness in the vessel wall unrelated to renal artery stenosis. Most congenital arteriovenous malformations present in the third or fourth decades of life. Post-traumatic fistulae often resolve spontaneously.

46
Anomalies of the Ureter
Howard M. Snyder III

1.   An ectopic ureterocele is most commonly associated with:

a.   urinary tract infections.
b.   urinary incontinence.
c.   poorly visualized upper collecting system of a complete duplication.
d.   poorly visualized lower collecting system of a complete duplication.
e.   bladder outlet obstruction.

Correct Answer: c   Reference Page: 2220
Rationale: In complete ureteral duplications with either ureteroceles or an ectopic ureter associated with the upper moiety, there is a greater likelihood of dysplastic nonfunctioning parenchyma with more distally ectopic locations of the ureteric orifice. Accordingly, an ectopic ureterocele which by definition is one extending down into the urethra below the bladder neck would be expected to have very poor visualization of the upper pole moiety.

2.   A 3-year-old child with a duplicated collecting system is found to have high pressure reflux upon voiding to the upper renal segment. The most appropriate statement is:

a.   this type of anomaly is commonly bilateral.
b.   the ureter to the upper segment is probably ectopic.
c.   the ureter to the lower segment is probably ectopic.
d.   the ureter to the lower segment is probably obstructed.
e.   reflux to the upper system occurs frequently with complete ureteral duplication.

Correct Answer: b   Reference Page: 2221-2222
Rationale: Reflux into an ectopic ureter occurs because there is a direct penetration of the ectopic ureter through the bladder neck or urethra without a submucosal tunnel. These ureters exhibit the paradox of being both obstructed and refluxing. The serial voiding VCUG is useful in making the diagnosis. Surgical intervention is the preferred management as with time there is no improvement in the anatomic abnormality.

3.   According to the Mackie and Stephens' theory of ureteral bud anomalies and their relationship to renal morphology, a ureteral bud which takes origin higher than normal on the mesonephric duct is likely to be associated with an element of renal dysplasia and:

a.   vesicoureteral reflux.
b.   distal ectopia.
c.   obstruction at ureterovesical junction.
d.   contralateral ureteral anomalies.
e.   poorly formed bladder-neck on ipsilateral side.

Correct Answer: b   Reference Page: 2202

Rationale: A higher-than-normal origin of the ureteral bud will lead to a shorter period of lateral migration of the ureter in the portion of the urogenital sinus to become the bladder, resulting in distal ectopia. In a duplicated system, the ureter to the lower pole enters the bladder in a higher position than the ureter to the upper pole.

4.   In a patient with complete duplication of the collecting system, cystoscopy classically reveals the upper pole orifice to be:

a.   lateral and caudad to the lower pole orifice.
b.   medial and caudad to the lower pole orifice.
c.   lateral and cephalad to the lower pole orifice.
d.   medial and cephalad to the lower pole orifice.
e.   distal to the bladder neck.

Correct Answer: b   Reference Page: 2200

Rationale: In complete ureteral duplication, the upper segment ureter arises more cephalad on the mesonephric duct than the lower segment ureter. However, because of differential growth of the urogenital sinus and earlier absorption of the lower ureter into the developing bladder, the lower segment ureter migrates more laterally and cephalad on the trigone than does the upper segment ureter—the Weigert-Meyer law.

47
The Wide Ureter

Stuart S. Howards and H. Norman Noe

1. **The standard classification of megaureters is which of the following?**

    a.   Primary and secondary obstructed ureter
    b.   Primary and secondary refluxing ureter
    c.   Refluxing and obstructed ureter
    d.   Refluxing, obstructed and nonrefluxing, nonobstructed ureter
    e.   Refluxing, obstructed, and adynamic ureter

Correct Answer: d   Reference Page: 2234

Rationale: The standard classification of megaureter is refluxing obstructed and nonrefluxing nonobstructed ureter. Secondary categories are primary and secondary of each of the above types. Nonrefluxing nonobstructed refers to all dilated ureters in which the VCUG and evaluation for obstruction are negative. It is a "wastebasket" category.

2. **Excluding the UPJ the most common site of congenital ureteral strictures is:**

    a.   isolated proximal ureter.
    b.   isolated mid-ureter.
    c.   isolated distal ureter.
    d.   combined mid- and distal ureter
    e.   combined proximal and distal ureter

Correct Answer: c   Reference Page: 2242

Rationale: The most common site of ureteral stricture is at the UPJ junction. However, when the stricture is in the ureter itself, by far the most common site is in the distal ureter. The other sites are very unusual.

3. **The most common cause of an obstructed megaureter is:**

    a.   congenital stricture.
    b.   crossing vessel.
    c.   idiopathic.
    d.   valves.
    e.   adynamic segment.

Correct Answer: e   Reference Page: 2243

Rationale: The adynamic segment is by far the most common cause of an obstructed megaureter. Congenital strictures are uncommon. Crossing vessels are controversial but probably occasionally cause obstruction. Valves are extremely rare.

4. **Excisional tailoring of a megaureter should be done with:**

    a. medial excision and tapering over a 16 F catheter.
    b. lateral excision and tapering over a 12 F catheter.
    c. medial excision and tapering over a 14 F catheter.
    d. lateral excision and tapering over an 8 F catheter.
    e. medial excision and tapering over an 8 F catheter.

Correct Answer: b   Reference Page: 2253

Rationale: The ureter should be excised laterally to preserve the medial blood supply and tapered over a 12 F catheter. A 16 F catheter would create too large a ureter, and an 8 F could be complicated by too narrow a remnant and obstruction.

5. **Repair of a megaureter with the technique of Kalinski or Starr has the advantage over the excision technique of:**

    a. decreased incidence of reflux.
    b. better results with large bulky ureters.
    c. shorter operating time.
    d. preserving blood supply.
    e. reducing extravesical dissection.

Correct Answer: d   Reference Page: 2254

Rationale: The main advantage of the Kalinski or Starr plication is that the blood supply is preserved, and thus fibrosis from ischemia is avoided. The results with large bulky ureters are actually not as good with the plication technique.

6. **Patients with megaureters should be evaluated with:**

    a. IVP and VCUG.
    b. sonogram and IVP.
    c. VCUG and pressure flow studies.
    d. pressure flow studies and a diuretic renogram.
    e. VCUG and a diuretic renogram.

Correct Answer: e   Reference Page: 2256

Rationale: Patients with a megaureter are almost invariably initially discovered with a sonogram or perhaps an IVP. However, to evaluate reflux a VCUG is essential and the most practical method for evaluating obstruction is a diuretic renogram. The pressure flow studies should be reserved for special situations.

7.   **The primary cause of an adynamic megaureter is:**

   a.   abnormal innervation.
   b.   obstruction or fibrosis.
   c.   disruption of muscular continuity.
   d.   tortuosity of the ureter.
   e.   absent and/or abnormal ganglia.

Correct Answer: c   Reference Page: 2246

Rationale: There have been many hypotheses about the cause of the adynamic ureter. However, the bulk of work suggests that obstruction of muscular continuity is the etiology.

48
Vesicoureteral Reflux and
Urinary Tract Infection in Children
R. Dixon Walker

1. **Which condition in a four-month-old male with urinary tract infection is most strongly associated with the development of a new renal scar?**

    a. uncircumcised status
    b. meatal stenosis
    c. dysfunctional voiding
    d. renal dysplasia
    e. Grade IV reflux

    Correct Answer: e   Reference Page: 2260
    Rationale: Grade IV reflux provides the greatest risk factor for renal scarring. Physiologic phimosis may predispose to UTI but not necessarily to renal scarring. Meatal stenosis is rare in infants and dysfunctional voiding occurs mostly as children learn voiding control. Renal dysplasia is congenital and not acquired.

2. **An eight-month-old girl with bilateral Grade IV reflux and a history of three urinary tract infections is most likely to have presented with:**

    a. diarrhea and vomiting.
    b. abdominal pain.
    c. symptoms of bladder irritability.
    d. failure to thrive and fever.
    e. hypertension.

    Correct Answer: d   Reference Page: 2261
    Rationale: Failure to thrive and fever are the two most common presentations of infants with complicated UTI. Diarrhea and vomiting occur less frequently. Bladder irritability, abdominal pain and hypertension would be presentations in an older child.

3. **A 4-year-old girl with unilateral Grade III reflux has a 1-year-old male sibling. Which screening test is most appropriate to rule out an inherited anomaly?**

    a. Voiding cystourethrogram
    b. Ultrasound
    c. Intravenous urogram
    d. DPTA renal scan
    e. DMSA renal scan

Correct Answer: a   Reference Page: 2267
Rationale: Jerkins and Noe found that 33% of siblings of patients with reflux also had reflux. A contrast or nuclear cystogram would be required to make the diagnosis. US will only suggest reflux 30–40% of the time.

4.   **Nuclear cystography has which advantage over contrast cystourethrography?**

    a.   Decreased discomfort for patient
    b.   Decreased cost for family
    c.   Decreased radiation dosage for patient
    d.   Increased visualization of associated abnormalities
    e.   Allows more precise grading

Correct Answer: c   Reference Page: 2263
Rationale: Majd and Belman (1979) indicated that the one clear advantage of nuclear cystography is decreased radiation. The discomfort to the patient is the same for both studies and contrast VCUG allows more precise grading and better visualization of associated abnormalities.

5.   **Which study will most precisely define renal damage resulting from Grade III unilateral reflux and a febrile urinary tract infection?**

    a.   Ultrasound
    b.   Intravenous urogram
    c.   DPTA renal scan
    d.   DMSA renal scan
    e.   CAT scan

Correct Answer: d   Reference Pages: 2263, 2269
Rationale: Rushton and Majd (1992) reviewed an extensive array of studies and found the DMSA renal scan was the most sensitive method to detect renal scarring.

6.   **A 10-year-old girl has persistent asymptomatic bacteriuria, bilateral Grade III reflux that has been surgically corrected, bilateral renal scarring on DMSA renal scan, 2+ proteinuria on dip stick urinalysis and a serum creatinine of 0.5 mg/dl. Which of the above is most directly related to eventual hypertension?**

    a.   Bacteriuria
    b.   Reflux
    c.   Renal scarring
    d.   Serum creatinine
    e.   Proteinuria

Correct Answer: c   Reference Page: 2274
Rationale: Bilateral renal scarring is the factor most directly related to hypertension. Reflux and bacteriuria are secondary factors.

7.   **Which factor is most characteristic of Grade I reflux in a 2-year-old girl?**

    a.   Will usually disappear spontaneously
    b.   Often associated with renal scarring
    c.   Usually requires surgical intervention
    d.   Is best diagnosed with nuclear cystography
    e.   May be improved with urethral dilation

Correct Answer: a   Reference Page: 2275
Rationale: Low grade reflux almost always resolves spontaneously and surgery is rarely indicated. There is little chance of damage to the kidney and urethral dilation has no place in the management.

8.   **A 2-year-old male with unilateral Grade III reflux, diagnosed after sibling screening, has no history of UTI. After 2 additional years of medical management what is the most likely effect on his refluxing kidney?**

    a.   Parenchymal thinning
    b.   Parenchymal scarring
    c.   Calyectesis
    d.   Decrease in GFR
    e.   No change

Correct Answer: e   Reference Pages: 2272, 2275
Rationale: Long-term sterile reflux of mid grade is unlikely to cause any change in the kidney over a short period of follow-up. This is a major factor that allows us to follow patients medically.

9.   **A 4-year-old girl with febrile UTI is found to have left Grade V reflux. DMSA scan shows 30% function in a scarred left kidney. The most appropriate management would be:**

    a.   antibacterials, urine cultures, repeat VCUG 6 months.
    b.   cutaneous vesicostomy.
    c.   cutaneous ureterostomy.
    d.   ureteral reimplantation.
    e.   nephrectomy.

Correct Answer: d   Reference Page: 2275

Rationale: Grade V reflux is very unlikely to resolve and there is already significant damage to the left kidney. Even though the kidney has only 30% of function it is worth salvaging and the most appropriate therapy would be ureteral reimplantation with or without tapering.

10. **A temporary complication which occurs in about 16% of patients after bilateral extravesical reimplantation is:**

  a. hydronephrosis.
  b. persistent reflux.
  c. severe dysuria.
  d. urinary retention.
  e. fever.

Correct Answer: d   Reference Page: 2279

Rationale: Urinary retention, often requiring clean intermittent catheterization, occurs in about 16% of patients after a Lich–Gregoire repair.

49
Prune Belly Syndrome

Douglas E. Coplen, Brent W. Snow, John W. Duckett

1. **Even though many men with a history of bilateral undescended testicles are fertile, there has never been a case of documented fertility in a patient with prune belly syndrome. The most likely explanation for this is that:**

   a. corporal and urethral abnormalities result in abnormal sexual function.
   b. testes in prune belly syndrome do not have normal germ cells.
   c. division of the blood vessels at the time of orchiopexy damages the testicle.
   d. prostatic and bladder neck abnormalities result in scant seminal emission.
   e. epididymal and vasal abnormalities do not allow sperm transport.

   Correct Answer: d   Reference Pages: 2300, 2305, 2310

   Rationale: Histologic evaluation of testes in patients with PBS reveals identical germ cell counts when compared to age matched controls with intraabdominal testes. While corporal, urethral, and testicular appendage abnormalities do exist in PBS patients, this would not explain infertility in all patients. Division of the testicular blood supply is not required for orchiopexy in all patients and is not necessarily associated with germ cell loss. The prostate and bladder neck are abnormal in all patients with PBS and this is most likely responsible for infertility in all patients.

2. **The best theory that accounts for the urologic manifestations of the prune belly syndrome is:**

   a. autosomal dominant genetic inheritance.
   b. early, transient urethral obstruction in the developing urinary tract.
   c. abnormality of the lateral plate mesoderm.
   d. retained yolk sac.
   e. primary urinary tract muscular abnormality.

   Correct Answer: b   Reference Page: 2298-2300

   Rationale: There is no single theory that best explains all of the manifestations of prune belly syndrome. There does not appear to be a genetic linkage. The bladder dilation and hydronephrosis are best explained by a transient infravesical obstruction since the mesodermal theory would not explain the absence of proximal hydronephrosis and the variable histologic picture in the bladders of PBS patients. Some experimental models of urethral obstruction have reproduced the PBS manifestations.

3.   **The term _pseudo-prune belly_ refers to:**

    a.   female patients with the typical abdominal wall defect.
    b.   prenatal hydroureteronephrosis and bladder distension that resolves.
    c.   typical prune belly appearance with urethral valves.
    d.   normal urinary tract with cryptorchidism and abnormal abdominal wall.
    e.   a patient lacking either the abdominal wall defect or bilateral cryptorchidism as components to PBS.

Correct Answer: e   Reference Page: 2312

Rationale: The urinary tract and abdominal wall changes of PBS have been found in female patients. In addition, the urinary tract deformations and undescended testicles can be found in the presence of a relatively normal abdominal wall. The management of the "pseudoprune" patient should be similar to that of the typical prune belly case since all of the urologic features and morbidity of the complete syndrome can occur.

4.   **The degree of renal dysplasia in patients with prune belly syndrome:**

    a.   is related to the degree of abdominal wall laxity and urinary tract dilation.
    b.   usually results in end-stage renal disease.
    c.   is reversible with early intervention.
    d.   is the most important factor influencing patient prognosis.
    e.   can be diagnosed with prenatal ultrasound.

Correct Answer: d   Reference Page: 2300, 2302, 2310

Rationale: Some prune belly patients are stillborn or die in the neonatal period with renal dysplasia and pulmonary hypoplasia. An additional 20% to 30% will later develop renal insufficiency. These patients cannot be reproducibly diagnosed antenatally and there is no evidence that early intervention alters the course of renal development. While many organ systems are affected in the prune belly syndrome, the degree of renal dysplasia most influences prognosis and outcome.

5.   **In the past, a child born with prune belly syndrome had a poor prognosis. Now, the majority have sufficient renal and pulmonary reserve to survive. The best initial urinary tract management to assure adequate urinary drainage and reduce stasis in most patients is:**

    a.   cutaneous vesicostomy.
    b.   complete reconstruction.
    c.   intermittent catheterization.
    d.   bladder massage.
    e.   loop ureterostomy.

Correct Answer: d   Reference Page: 2306-2307

Rationale: Adequate urinary drainage to reduce stasis and infection is the critical factor in the treatment of the child with PBS. Unlike posterior urethral valves, PBS is low pressure and nonobstructive and the reflux in the absence of infection will not result in renal damage. Catheter drainage should be discouraged since infection will result. Upper tract urinary diversion is rarely required in the absence of obstruction. In cases of urethral atresia or inadequate bladder emptying with massage, cutaneous vesicostomy is indicated. While complete reconstruction improves the radiographic appearance of the urinary tract it does not necessarily improve drainage.

6. **The bladder of the patient with prune belly syndrome is usually very large. The function is best characterized as:**

a. being a contractile flaccid sensory neurogenic bladder.
b. a non-neurogenic neurogenic bladder with high voiding pressures.
c. a normally synergistic bladder with a shift in the manometric curve to the right.
d. a contractile bladder with myogenic failure.
e. a high pressure bladder with fixed outlet resistance.

Correct Answer: c   Reference Page: 2302, 2303, 2307

Rationale: The PBS bladder is capacious. Many patients have significant postvoid-residual urine volumes suggesting an altered state of unbalanced voiding dynamics. However, urodynamic evaluation has not demonstrated anatomic or functional evidence of bladder outlet obstruction. The large bladder capacity shifts the cystometry curve to the right. Reduction cystoplasty has been utilized by some, but whether a smaller bladder increases detrusor efficiency is unclear. External sphincterotomy appears to be the most successful treatment for balance voiding.

7. **Management of the urinary tract in prune belly syndrome can be either a "conservative" observational approach or an "aggressive" reconstructive approach. Based on the Children's Hospital of Philadelphia experience which of the following statements is true?**

a. Vesicoureteral reflux usually requires surgical treatment.
b. Long-term outcomes are the same regardless of the initial management approach.
c. Temporary urinary diversion is required more than half the time.
d. Abdominal wall reconstruction improves urinary tract dynamics.
e. Ureteral reconstruction is eventually required for adequate peristalsis.

Correct Answer: b   Reference Page: 2311-2312

Rationale: The refluxing and dilated ureter in PBS rarely requires reconstruction unless recurrent infections are a problem. These reconstructions are technically difficult and associated with a high complication rate. Usually, a combination of preventive antibiotics and vigilant observation to assure that the urinary tract does not decompensate are sufficient in over 50% of patients. This conservative approach is not associated with a higher incidence of renal insufficiency or ESRD when compared to series where aggressive reconstruction was performed early in management.

50
Principals of Pediatric Urinary Tract Reconstruction

Curtis A. Sheldon and Howard M. Snyder III

1. **Which statement accurately reflects the association of urointestinal anastomoses and subsequent malignancy?**

   a. Risk is eliminated following urine diversion away from anastomosis.
   b. Risk is minimal if malignancy is not evident by 10 years.
   c. An intact fecal stream is required to generate malignancy.
   d. When undiverting a ureterosigmoidostomy, the anastomoses should be excised.
   e. Malignancies have not been reported following ileocystoplasty or colocystoplasty for benign bladder disease.

   Correct Answer: d　　　Reference Page: 2323

   Rationale: The mean interval between ureterosigmoidostomy and presentation of malignancy is 24 years. Because malignancy has been reported in augmented bladder for benign disease, an intact fecal stream is not an absolute prerequisite. Malignancy developing at the site of ureteral stumps following defunctionalization of the ureterosigmoidostomy accounts for approximately 17% of all ureterosigmoidostomy related malignancies. Accordingly, such stumps should be entirely excised.

2. **Bladder augmentation is performed in order to decrease bladder pressure and increase capacity. What statement most accurately reflects the physiologic principles regarding this process?**

   a. Within the wall of an augmented bladder, wall tension is universally equally distributed.
   b. Within the lumen of an augmented bladder, the pressure is greatest in the portion composed of native bladder.
   c. The width of the augmenting intestinal segment is less important in determining ultimate capacity than is the length.
   d. Detubularization geometrically enhances the capacity but does not significantly influence muscular contraction.
   e. The degree to which the bladder is opened also contributes to ultimate outcome.

   Correct Answer: e　　　Reference Page: 2330

   Rationale: Detubularization is a critical component of intestinocystoplasty which both enhances capacity geometrically and interrupts peristalsis by dividing circular muscle fibers. The bladder should be prepared by a generous "clam cystoplasty" incision. Pressure is equally distributed throughout the augmented bladder whereas wall tension is greatest in those portions of the bladder associated with the greatest radius of curvature.

3.	**True statements regarding the Mitrofanoff continent, catheterizable neourethra include all of the following *except*:**

    a.	it may be exteriorized to the lower abdominal wall, umbilicus or perineum.
    b.	it may be implanted into the native bladder.
    c.	luminal incontinence is a common complication.
    d.	the greatest risk is stomal stenosis.
    e.	it may be implanted into the gastric or colonic segment of an augmented bladder.

Correct Answer: c   Reference Page:

Rationale: The Mitrofanoff neourethra is a highly successful and versatile procedure to allow continent catheter access to the urinary bladder. The continence rate is 96%. However, the incidence of stomal stenosis is approximately 13%. It may be implanted into native bladder, stomach, or colon with excellent success.

4.	**A 14-year-old female who had an ileocystoplasty 2 years previously presents with nausea, bilious emesis, fever, and abdominal pain. The abdomen is distended and tender to palpation. Flat and upright radiographs of the abdomen reveal a nonspecific gas pattern. A cystogram reveals no evidence of perforation. Which statement accurately reflects this patient's situation?**

    a.	Absence of air-fluid levels excludes bowel obstruction.
    b.	Absence of extravasation excludes bladder perforation.
    c.	Bladder perforation carries a low morbidity.
    d.	Bladder perforation remains a significant concern for this patient.
    e.	She should be treated for pyelonephritis.

Correct Answer: d   Reference Page: 2390

Rationale: Spontaneous rupture of the bladder is a life-threatening complication of augmentation which may occur late following augmentation and may not be diagnosed by cystography. Aggressive management is indicated and consideration should be given to early laparotomy.

5.   An 8-year-old male presents with lethargy and vomiting and is found to have systemic acidosis 4 months following colocystoplasty. True statements regarding this condition include all of the following *except*:

a.   Azotemia is a risk factor.
b.   Acidosis is avoidable by employing ileum.
c.   Acidosis is potentiated by a large surface of intestinal tissue.
d.   Acidosis may contribute to diminished somatic growth.
e.   Gastrocystoplasty, ureterocystoplasty, and autoaugmentation are protective of acidosis in azotemia.

Correct Answer: b   Reference Page: 2319
Rationale: Systemic acidosis can occur with exposure of urine to colonic, jejunal or ileal surfaces. It is potentiated by azotemia and large surface area. Acidosis in children is associated with blunted statural growth. Gastrocystoplasty excretes acid while ureterocystoplasty and autoaugmentation are metabolically inert.

6.   A 7-year-old female is referred following previous reconstruction for bladder exstrophy which included a Young-Dees-Leadbetter bladder neck reconstruction. She is totally incontinent of urine despite a trial of oxybutynin hydrochloride and intermittent catheterization. Evaluation reveals an incompetent bladder outlet and she is scheduled for revision of her bladder outlet. What finding would suggest that concomitant augmentation is *not* necessary?

a.   Compliance at capacity of 2.5 ml/cm H_2O
b.   Bladder capacity of 140 ml
c.   Absence of vesicoureteral reflux
d.   Leak point pressure less than 40 cm H_2O
e.   Absence of bacteria

Correct Answer: a   Reference Page: 2362
Rationale: Failure to augment an anticholinergic-resistant high pressure bladder is a common cause of failure of bladder outlet reconstruction. Conversely, the bladder's capacity and compliance are difficult to assess due to a lack of incentive to gain capacity from absent bladder outlet resistance. A bladder capacity exceeding 60% expected for age or if lower capacity, a compliance at capacity exceeding 2 ml/cm H_2O is suggestive that augmentation may not be necessary.

7.   A 12-year-old male with myelodysplasia is referred for progressive hydronephrosis, recurrent urinary tract infection and incontinence. Urodynamic
evaluation reveals a high pressure, low capacity bladder unresponsive to
oxybutynin chloride therapy. Bladder augmentation is scheduled. Which of the
following parameters would suggest that concomitant bladder outlet reconstruction is necessary?

a.   A urethral pressure profile maximum of 60 cm H_2O
b.   A leak point pressure of 60 cm H_2O
c.   A stress leak point pressure of 60 cm H_2O
d.   A closed bladder outlet on upright cystography
e.   Striated sphincter innervation documented by EMG

Correct Answer: c   Reference Page: 2330

Rationale: While stress leak point pressure appears to be a reliable indication of
bladder outlet competency, urethral pressure profilemetry and leak point pressure have
been less reliable. A closed bladder neck on upright cystography and EMG have also
proven useful in myelodysplasia.

51
Urethral Lesions in Infants and Children
Grahame H.H. Smith and John W. Duckett

1. **When ablating a posterior urethral valve, it is best to:**

   a. resect it completely using a loop electrode and a cutting current.
   b. incise it at 12 o'clock using a cutting current.
   c. ablate it completely with a flexible electrode and a coagulating current.
   d. use a crochet hook to engage the valve with radiologic control.
   e. wait until the child is over 3 months of age.

   Correct Answer: b   Reference Page: 2423
   Rationale: a. Is wrong. Resecting the valve completely with a loop will usually result in a stricture. b. Is correct. Incising the valve at 12 o'clock or at 5 and 7 o'clock will relieve the obstruction. The residual leaflets do not matter. c. Is wrong. A coagulating current should not be used. Short bursts of cutting current should be utilized. d. Is wrong. The hook must be properly insulated or the urethra will be damaged. e. Is wrong. Modern endoscopes can be used to safely ablate a PUV in the newborn period.

2. **A vesicostomy should be performed for a patient with posterior urethral valves if:**

   a. renal failure worsens.
   b. the valve cannot be ablated in a satisfactory manner.
   c. the patient presents in the newborn period.
   d. there is not a rapid fall in creatinine after valve ablation.
   e. the patient is septic.

   Correct Answer: b   Reference Page: 2423
   Rationale: a. Is wrong. Renal failure may worsen for several reasons, including infection, obstruction, full valve bladder syndrome and hyperfiltration injury. The cause of deterioration should be determined before treatment is undertaken. b. Is correct. If valve ablation cannot be performed because of technical difficulties then a vesicostomy is the best form of temporary diversion. c. Is wrong. Modern endoscopes allow safe valve ablation in the newborn period. d. Is wrong. We allow several weeks for the creatinine to fall before deciding to perform a vesicostomy. e. Is wrong. Sepsis can be initially treated with antibiotics and feeding tube drainage of the bladder.

3. **CMJs or corticomedullary junctions seen on renal ultrasound indicate:**

a. a good prognosis.
b. a poor prognosis.
c. calcification of the medulla.
d. dysplasia.
e. a technically satisfactory study.

Correct Answer: a   Reference Page: 2419
Rationale: a. Is correct. In 28 infants with PUV reported by Hulbert et. al, 1992, adequate renal function was present in 17 of 17 infants with CMJs seen on ultrasound. b. Is wrong. c. Is wrong. Calcification of the medulla results in increased echogenicity and decreased corticomedullary differentiation. d. Is wrong. Loss of CMJs is associated with dysplasia e. Is wrong. The study can be technically satisfactory but if the kidneys are severely damaged, no CMJs will be seen. CMJs are not seen in older children and adults.

4. **In utero treatment of posterior urethral valves:**

a. reduces the incidence of end stage renal failure.
b. reduces infant mortality.
c. has been made possible by accurate prenatal ultrasound diagnosis.
d. is still controversial and experimental.
e. reduces the incidence of sepsis in newborns with valves.

Correct Answer: d   Reference Page: 2421
Rationale: a. Is wrong. There is no evidence for this at present. b. Is wrong. There is no evidence for this at present. c. Is wrong. It is difficult to accurately identify the cause of bilateral hydronephrosis picked up by antenatal ultrasound. The differential diagnosis includes prune belly syndrome, bilateral high grade reflux and bilateral megaureters. d. Is correct. The treatment is experimental and should only be performed in a research fetal center. e. Is wrong. There is no evidence for this at present.

5. **The VURD syndrome in patients with posterior urethral valves:**

a. stands for *V*esico*U*reteric *R*eflux and *D*ysplasia.
b. is of little consequence to the practicing urologist.
c. can be cured by nephrectomy.
d. is associated with a worse prognosis.
e. is associated with spurious renal function on an IVP.

Correct Answer: e   Reference Page: 2425
Rationale: a. Is wrong. It stands for *v*alve, *u*nilateral *r*eflux and *d*ysplasia. b. Is wrong. A physician unaware of the syndrome may see spurious renal function on IVP and this may lead to ureteric reimplantation of a nonfunctioning kidney. c. Is wrong. The syndrome is diagnosed at the time of presentation and the patient will always have this label. The refluxing unit acts as a pop-off mechanism to protect the other kidney; removing it prematurely may be unwise. d. Is wrong. The prognosis is improved in patients with the VURD syndrome. e. Is correct. This is due to reflux of contrast from the bladder into the nonfunctioning collecting system.

6.   **Urethral prolapse in childhood:**

a.   should be treated by circumferential resection, after the diagnosis is confirmed by cystoscopy.
b.   may mimic a rhabdomyosarcoma of the vagina.
c.   is less common than urethral prolapse during middle age.
d.   is suggestive of sexual abuse.
e.   is a condition that requires urgent treatment.

Correct Answer: b   Reference Page: 2436
Rationale: a. Is wrong. It should be initially treated by estrogen cream and sitz baths. b.Is correct. c. Is wrong. It occurs in the young and the old. d. Is wrong. There is no evidence for this. e. Is wrong. It is a mucosal prolapse only and should be initially treated conservatively.

7.   **A valve of Guerin or lacuna magna:**

a.   is associated with urethral obstruction.
b.   is a common embryological variant, usually asymptomatic.
c.   should be treated by cystoscopic ablation.
d.   is a cause of recurrent urinary tract infections.
e.   is best diagnosed by cystoscopy.

Correct Answer: b   Reference Page: 2435
Rationale: a. Is wrong. It may cause turbulence of urinary flow at the meatus, but is not usually obstructive. b. Is correct. It has been reported in 50% of routine postmortems. c. Is wrong. It should only be treated if symptomatic, and in that case by incising with sharp scissors. d. Is wrong. There is no evidence for this. It may cause hematuria or dysuria. e. Is wrong. It is best diagnosed by probing the fossa navicularis with a blunt needle or lacrimal probe.

8. **When treating patients with posterior urethral valves, high loop ureterostomy diversion:**

    a.   is best reserved for patients in whom the valve cannot be ablated.
    b.   is a superior treatment to valve ablation in the newborn period.
    c.   is easy to perform and to reverse.
    d.   has been replaced by low loop ureterostomy.
    e.   is a controversial treatment.

Correct Answer: e   Reference Page: 2424

Rationale: a. Is wrong. Vesicostomy is a better option. b. Is wrong. There is no good evidence for this and even Churchill (1990) recommends valve ablation initially. c. Is wrong. It may be easy to perform, but it is difficult to reverse. d. Is wrong. Low loop ureterostomy should not be used because of the difficulty with reconstruction. Ureteric reimplantation into the PUV bladder is required and this has a high incidence of complications. e. Is correct. Churchill (1990) believes that high diversion should still be used for neonates that do not respond to valve ablation. We strongly disagree and recommend vesicostomy.

52

Anomalies of the Bladder and Cloaca

Douglas A. Canning, Harry P. Koo, John W. Duckett

1. **A newborn male is referred with a suspected epispadias. He has a small urethral meatus at the tip of his penis. He has a second meatus at the penopubic junction. Ultrasound examination is suspicious for two bladders, one anterior to the other. Two normal kidneys exist. IVP shows that the two kidneys empty via normal ureters into the posterior bladder which appears normal. Treatment should include:**

   a. posterior iliac osteotomy to provide closure of the pubic ring and reconstruction of the epispadiac urethra.
   b. removal of the anterior bladder, bladder neck and urethra.
   c. removal of the septum between both bladders to create one large bladder.
   d. removal of the anterior bladder at age 6 to 12 months and preservation of the epispadiac urethral meatus.
   e. observation for development of symptoms.

   Correct Answer: d   Reference Page: 2447

   Rationale: Duplication with epispadias is rare, but reported. Treatment should be individualized. There is no need to preserve the anterior bladder here. It subtends no functioning renal tissue. Closure with osteotomy is used to improve continence and is not necessary in a continent urethra. Removal of the anterior bladder is desirable to reduce risk of pyocystis in a nonfunctioning bladder. There may be functioning prostate tissue at the bladder neck which should be preserved. Removal of the bladder neck and the epispadiac urethra is difficult surgery that risks injury to ejaculation and erection and may result in cyst formation if all glandular tissue is not removed. There is no indication to enlarge the posterior bladder. Observation may be attempted, but in most cases removal of the accessory bladder will be necessary.

2.   **A newborn is referred with a persistent wet umbilicus. The area around the umbilicus is reddened but not irritated. The child has normal kidneys and bladder on ultrasound and no cyst is seen superior to the bladder. The retrograde fistulogram demonstrates an irregular tract to the dome of the bladder but not entering the bladder. Voiding cystourethrogram is normal. The next step is to:**

    a.   perform cystoscopy to identify the opening into the fistula.
    b.   explore the fistula and marsupialize it.
    c.   explore the fistula and remove it with a cuff of bladder and the umbilicus.
    d.   remove the fistula with a cuff of bladder.
    e.   observe.

Correct Answer: d   Reference Page: 2452

Rationale: Cystoscopy is rarely helpful in identifying the site of the fistula. Marsupialization will do nothing but worsen drainage from the small fistula. It is not necessary to remove the umbilicus. Observation presumes the fistula will close. If it closes, the child is still left with the fistula tract and a possible cyst. The fistula should be removed with a cuff of bladder to avoid possibility of adenocarcinoma of the bladder dome later in life. The umbilicus should be preserved.

3.   **A healthy 26-year-old delivers a full-term baby at the obstetrical suite in your hospital. APGAR scores are normal. The pediatrician identifies the anomaly as bladder exstrophy, but is unsure of the sex of the child or what to do next. You are called in consultation. There is no visible bowel at the site of the bladder and a hemiscrotum is present adjacent to each side of the bladder. The penis is epispadiac. What should be done next?**

    a.   Order karyotype to help in sex assignment.
    b.   Obtain chest x-ray, complete blood count, serum blood urea nitrogen (BUN) and creatinine.
    c.   Obtain orthopedics consult to evaluate for hip dislocation.
    d.   Alert the operating room for immediate 5 hour bladder exstrophy closure.
    e.   Transport child to tertiary care center for bladder closure at age 12 to 24 hours.

Correct Answer: e   Reference Page: 2458-2461

Rationale: Sex assignment is based on physical exam, not karyotype. Only very rarely does a male child require sex reassignment in classic bladder exstrophy. The decision is based on size of the phallus, not on the genotype. All but the most rudimentary phallus can be reconstructed. Most infants with bladder exstrophy have normal lungs and routine chest x-ray is not indicated. BUN and creatinine reflect the mother's serum levels for the first 24 hours and provide no information at this early perinatal period. Although hip dysplasia is reported with exstrophy, it is rare. Consultation with an orthopedist is important only if pelvic osteotomy is contemplated. The child should not undergo closure of the bladder until stable and well hydrated. Usually the soonest this can be accomplished is at 18 to 24 hours.

4. **You are called to see an infant with bladder exstrophy who has undergone closure at two weeks of age with bilateral anterior iliac osteotomy. She has been hypertensive for the past 48 hours. On close examination you note weakness on dorsiflexion of the right great toe. The most appropriate management is:**

    a. obtain a plain film of the pelvis to assess the degree of pubic diastasis.
    b. release the external fixation device.
    c. reduce tension on the external fixation device and monitor blood pressure.
    d. perform ultrasound to look for evidence of hematoma at Alcock's canal.
    e. call neurosurgery for evaluation of suspected surgical injury to sciatic nerve.

Correct Answer: c   Reference Page: 2466

Rationale: Following closure of the bladder, the absolute degree of pubic diastasis is variable. Imaging the pelvis will not help in the management of this postoperative complication. Even if diastasis is recurrent, nothing should be done to provide closer approximation of the pelvis at this point. This child is suffering from the effects of overzealous compression of the external fixator. Too much medial rotation of the pelvis results in tension on the sciatic nerve that results in transient weakness and/or reflex induced vasoconstriction and subsequent hypertension. The external fixator need not be removed, but should be loosened. There is no need to suspect surgical injury to the nerve at this time.

5. **A 4-year-old boy has moved with his family to your area. He was born with classic bladder exstrophy and had a successful newborn closure at birth. He is totally incontinent in diapers. He is in preschool and his mother would like him to be dry. No other surgery has been performed. His abdominal scar is well healed to the level of the penopubic junction revealing a complete epispadias which is draining clear fluid. His kidneys are normal on ultrasound and the bladder measures approximately 30 cc in volume. There is moderate pubic diastasis on the plain film. What do you recommend next?**

    a. Bilateral anterior iliac osteotomy to provide better pubic approximation followed by Young-Dees-Leadbetter-Jeffs bladder neck reconstruction
    b. Epispadias repair
    c. Collagen injection at the bladder neck
    d. Ureterosigmoidostomy with cystectomy
    e. Bladder neck reconstruction

Correct Answer: b   Reference Page: 2467-2468

Rationale: Bladder neck reconstruction with or without osteotomy is much less successful if done before bladder size is adequate (60 cc). Epispadias repair has been shown to be effective at improving bladder volume during the incontinence period. Collagen injection may help a select group of patients improve bladder neck resistance in hopes of improving bladder volume prior to bladder neck reconstruction, but this rarely works prior to epispadias repair. Ureterosigmoidostomy or bladder augmentation should not be recommended until the bladder has failed to gain volume after epispadias repair.

6.   **A 21-year-old woman reports that she was born with bladder exstrophy. She is 18 weeks pregnant. Her bladder was closed at birth with bilateral posterior iliac osteotomy and the patient had been somewhat continent during the day, but leaked a bit at night. For this reason, she underwent augmentation cystoplasty at age 12 and now catheterizes every 6 hours through her native urethra. Her obstetrician would like your opinion on her urologic care during the pregnancy. Your recommendation should be to:**

a.   watch for difficulty with urethral catheterizations, increase frequency of catheterizations, full-term delivery with cesarean section.

b.   start prophylactic antibiotics, continue pregnancy until fetus viable for elective preterm vaginal delivery.

c.   obtain frequent renal ultrasounds to watch for maternal hydronephrosis, start prophylactic antibiotics, increase frequency of catheterizations.

d.   start prophylactic antibiotics, continue pregnancy to term, vaginal delivery.

e.   watch for difficulty with urethral catheterizations, elective pre-term vaginal delivery.

Correct Answer: a   Reference Page: 2483

Rationale: In the absence of infection there is no need to initiate prophylactic antibiotics, even if the patient is catheterizing to drain an augmented bladder. The patient should be catheterizing frequently enough to prevent stasis and colonization of bacteria, if possible every 4 to 6 hours. There is no reason to deliver the baby early unless complications develop during the pregnancy. Exstrophy patients, with very few exceptions, should deliver via cesarean section to prevent injury to the pelvic reconstruction. A number of women with exstrophy will develop difficulty with catheterization as the uterus enlarges late in pregnancy.

7.   **An 11-month-old female with a cloaca anomaly is on the pediatric ward with recurrent febrile breakthrough urinary tract infections despite antibiotic prophylaxis. Her VCUG shows grade II vesicoureteral reflux bilaterally with good bladder emptying. She had loop colostomy performed as a newborn and is awaiting definitive repair of her anus through a posterior sagittal approach. Renal ultrasound is normal. You recommend:**

a.   vesicostomy.
b.   intermittent catheterization.
c.   bilateral ureteral reimplantation.
d.   rotate antibiotic prophylaxis between nitrofurantoin, sulfamethoxazole-trimetho-prim, and amoxicillin.
e.   revision of loop colostomy to divided colostomy.

Correct Answer: e   Reference Page: 2489

Rationale: A divided colostomy prevents contamination of the genitourinary tract with feces. This infant, with bilateral vesicoureteric reflux is particularly at risk. Performing vesicostomy would reduce the tendency to reflux, but would not address the fecal contamination. Bilateral reimplantation would likewise fail to prevent contamination. Rotating the antibiotic prophylaxis is sometimes effective, but does not address the basic problem of the source of the contamination, the colon.

53

Myelomeningocele and Neuropathic Bladder
Mark F. Bellinger

1. **The most significant prognostic urodynamic factor in predicting the likelihood of upper urinary tract deterioration in children with myelodysplasia is:**

   a. the presence of uninhibited detrusor contraction.
   b. elevated postvoid residual urine volume.
   c. elevated leak point pressure.
   d. areflexic sphincter.
   e. decreased outlet resistance.

   Correct Answer: c   Reference Page: 2499
   Rationale: Elevated intravesical pressure may result from detrusor-external sphincter dyssynergy. Elevated leak point pressures may result in vesicoureteric reflux or hydronephrosis secondary to thickened bladder wall and high intramural tension.

2. **All of the following mechanisms are thought to play a role in the mechanism of transurethral electric bladder stimulation *except*:**

   a. stimulation of detrusor contraction.
   b. activation of mural receptors.
   c. vegetative afferentation.
   d. facilitation of efferent pathways.
   e. coordination of detrusor and sphincter activity.

   Correct Answer: e   Reference Page: 2512
   Rationale: Transurethral electrical bladder stimulation is thought to act by all of the above mechanisms except for coordination of detrusor/sphincter activity. The activation of mural receptors which have remained dormant (due to lack of afferent innervation) triggers detrusor contractions. Vegetative afferentation then proceeds, facilitating efferent pathways.

3. **Spontaneous bladder perforation after enterocystoplasty is most likely related to:**

   a. the presence of bladder calculi.
   b. ischemic necrosis.
   c. chronic inflammation.
   d. granulomatous cystitis.
   e. lack of bladder sensation.

   Correct Answer: b   Reference Page: 2503

Rationale: Ischemic necrosis of the augmented bladder wall may result from inefficient bladder emptying and chronic overdistension. Mucus plugs may play a role in chronic distension.

4.   **High-grade vesicoureteric reflux in a child with neurovesical dysfunction and detrusor/sphincter dyssynergia may be best managed initially by:**

a.   ureteral reimplantation.
b.   suprapubic cystostomy.
c.   subureteric (collagen, Teflon) injection therapy.
d.   intermittent catheterization and anticholinergic therapy.
e.   intermittent catheterization and phenylpropanolamine.

Correct Answer: d   Reference Page: 2499

Rationale: Intermittent catheterization combined with anticholinergic therapy or temporary urinary diversion by cutaneous vesicostomy may best initially decompress a high-pressure bladder. Antireflux procedures should not be considered until bladder pressures and emptying have been stabilized, at times requiring bladder augmentation.

5.   **The potential complications of colocystoplasty include all *except*:**

a.   calculus formation.
b.   neoplasia.
c.   diarrhea.
d.   spontaneous bladder rupture.
e.   metabolic alkalosis.

Correct Answer: e   Reference Page: 2505

Rationale: The net excretion of hydrogen and chloride into the urine from gastric segments may result in hypochloremic metabolic alkalosis after gastrocystoplasty.

6.   **Daytime urinary frequency in a child without urinary tract infection or neurological findings may best be managed by:**

a.   oxybutynin.
b.   imipramine.
c.   hypnosis.
d.   observation.
e.   psychotherapy.

Correct Answer: d   Reference Page: 2520

Rationale: Daytime urinary frequency is generally managed by benign neglect. In most instances, toileting changes, pharmacotherapy, and invasive therapy prove unsuccessful and may actually worsen symptoms.

7. **Asymptomatic urinary tract infection in a child without vesicoureteric reflux who is maintained on a regimen of intermittent catheterization is best managed by:**

    a. observation.
    b. prophylactic antibacterial therapy.
    c. bladder irrigation with antibiotic solution.
    d. monthly urine cultures and appropriate antibiotic therapy.
    e. discontinuation of intermittent catheterization.

Correct Answer: a   Reference Page: 2575

Rationale: Asymptomatic urinary tract infection in a child who does not have vesicoureteric reflux is best observed. Treatment may be indicated if infections become symptomatic, but overtreatment of asymptomatic infections may promote the growth of resistant organisms.

54

Genital Anomalies

Terry W. Hensle

1. **The most appropriate early treatment for the infant born with penile agenesis is:**

   a. early hypospadias repair.
   b. perineal urethrostomy.
   c. gonadectomy and gender reassignment.
   d. endocrine evaluation.
   e. insertion of a tissue expander for a penile reconstruction.

   Correct Answer: c   Reference Page: 2530
   Rationale: Congenital absence of the penis is a rare condition that probably results from failure of the genital tubricle to develop. Endocrine function in these patients has been shown to be normal as judged by a normal response to gonadotropin stimulation. The recommended treatment should be early gender reassignment and gonadectomy. The urethra should be transposed anteriorly away from the anal verge and the scrotal skin should be preserved to later aid vaginal construction.

2. **The embryologic origin of the upper portion of the vagina is from the:**

   a. Mesonephric duct.
   b. Wolffian duct.
   c. Mullerian duct.
   d. urogenital sinus.
   e. Gartners duct.

   Correct Answer: c   Reference Page: 2537
   Rationale: The exact embryologic origin of the vagina is not totally certain. It is most likely that the upper four fifths of the vagina is formed from the Mullerian duct and the lower fifth from the urogenital sinus.

3. **The most common genitourinary abnormality associated with vaginal atresia is:**

   a. renal agenesis.
   b. renal duplication.
   c. crossed fused ectopia.
   d. vesicoureteral reflux.
   e. UPJ obstruction.

Correct Answer: a   Reference Page: 2537
Rationale: The association between congenital absence of the vagina and anomalies of the genitourinary system is very common, approximately one-third of these patients will have renal abnormalities. The most common abnormality is agenesis of 1 kidney followed by ectopia of 1 or both kidneys.

4.   **Cloacal anomalies occur at 4 to 6 weeks of gestation due to:**

    a.   failure of the cloacal membrane to form.
    b.   failure of the urorectal septum to divide allantois and hindgut.
    c.   a fusion anomaly of the Mullerian ducts.
    d.   premature rupture of the urogenital sinus.
    e.   failure of the vaginal plate to develop.

Correct Answer: b   Reference Page: 2542
Rationale: At 4 to 6 weeks of gestation the urorectal septum should divide the allantois and hindgut. If this separation does not take place a common cloaca will result.

5.   **Urethral prolapse occurs most commonly in:**

    a.   oriental males.
    b.   caucasian females.
    c.   caucasian males.
    d.   black females.
    e.   black males.

Correct Answer: d   Reference Page: 2453
Rationale: Prolapse of the urethra occurs almost exclusively in black girls between the ages of 3 and 9 years. The child frequently has blood spotting on the underwear and a necrotic mass at the introitus which represents a prolapsed and infarcted portion of the anterior portion of the anterior urethra.

6.   **Microphallus is commonly associated with:**

    a.   hypospadias.
    b.   Klippel-Feil syndrome.
    c.   Prader-Willi syndrome.
    d.   bladder exstrophy.
    e.   Mayer-Rokitansky syndrome.

Correct Answer: c   Reference Page: 2532
Rationale: In general the etiology of microphallus is thought to be either inadequate androgen stimulation of the target organ or insensitivity of the target organ to

available androgen. There are a number of central defects where microphallus is a definable part of the syndrome including the Prader-Willi syndrome and Kallman syndrome.

7. **Penile duplication anomalies occur most frequently in patients with:**

a. true hermaphroditism.
b. bladder exstrophy.
c. meningomyelocele.
d. prune belly syndrome.
e. posterior urethral valves.

Correct Answer: b   Reference Page: 2531

Rationale: Duplication of the penis is a rare anomaly probably resulting from incomplete fusion of the genital tubricle. The anomaly appears in 2 basic forms. The first and more common being the bifid penis which is often associated with the exstrophy epispadias complex and is present in almost every male with cloacal exstrophy.

8. **Lateral curvature of the penis is usually caused by:**

a. circumcision injury.
b. an injury to 1 corporal body.
c. a foreshortened urethra.
d. overgrowth of 1 corporal body.
e. atresia of 1 corporal body.

Correct Answer: d   Reference Page: 2533

Rationale: Lateral penile curvature is usually recognized in early childhood and must be differentiated from chordee without hypospadias. Lateral curvature is usually caused by an overgrowth of 1 corporal body; however, the defect at times can be associated with a corporal injury and foreshortening of 1 corporal body. This is less frequent.

55
Hypospadias
Laurence Baskin and John W. Duckett

1. **In anterior hypospadias what factor is the most important in determining the repair technique?**

   a. Glans configuration
   b. Chordee
   c. Meatal size
   d. Quality of the ventral urethral skin
   e. Depth of the urethral pit

   Correct Answer: d   Reference Page: 2572

   Rationale: The quality of the skin of the ventral urethra is critical in deciding which hypospadias technique is most suitable. For example in some cases with a subcorneal meatus that has a thick ventral urethral skin, a MAGPI repair may be suitable whereas in other cases the ventral urethral skin is so thin that once it is excised to healthy urethra, the meatus may be quite proximal on the penile shaft (Figure 57-8B) requiring an onlay island flap repair.

2. **Buccal mucosa free grafts are most suitable for:**

   a. primary perineal hypospadias repairs where the prepuce is inadequate to bridge the necessary gap for the urethroplasty.
   b. in redo cases when local skin is unavailable for creation of a neourethra.
   c. tube urethroplasties.
   d. in epispadias.
   e. patch grafts in urethral stricture disease.

   Correct Answer: b   Reference Page: 2577

   Rationale: Buccal mucosa free grafts should only be used when local vascularized skin is not available for the neourethra. Typically this occurs in hypospadias or epispadias cases that have had multiple prior operations. Buccal mucosa free grafts work best as an onlay fashion when a healthy urethral plate can receive the graft. Buccal mucosa grafts have been successfully used for urethral stricture diseases; however, in general a vascularized penile skin flap is a better first choice than a free graft of any material.

3.   **Patients with penoscrotal transposition, proximal hypospadias and a nonpalpable testicle:**

a.   require orchiopexy at the time of the hypospadias repair.
b.   should have the orchiopexy performed at a separate operation so as not to interfere with the penoscrotal transposition correction.
c.   should have the penoscrotal transposition repaired at a separate operation so as not to interfere with the urethroplasty.
d.   can usually be managed in one operation.
e.   require an abdominal pelvic ultrasound preop.

Correct Answer: e   Reference Page: 2555
Rationale: Patients with a nonpalpable testicle and proximal hypospadias should be worked up for intersex. They require evaluation for female internal organs with a rectal exam and confirmation by pelvic ultrasound. A chromosome analysis will guide the differential diagnosis.

Patients with penoscrotal transposition and proximal hypospadias traditionally have the urethroplasty performed first followed by repair of the penoscrotal transposition 6-9 months after the first stage. Performing a single stage repair has the potential to violate the blood supply to the preputial skin flap urethroplasty.

4.   **During correction of penile curvature it is most appropriate to:**

a.   dissect under the urethral plate while still preserving the urethral plate to release chordee tissue.
b.   use absorbable sutures to prevent suture knots that will result from permanent material.
c.   incise through the tunica albuginea of the corpora cavernosa.
d.   place parallel plication sutures with excision of tunica tissue.
e.   perform deep cuts in the midline of the ventrum of the penis.

Correct Answer: c   Reference Page: 2560
Rationale: Penile curvature can be from skin and/or dartos fascia tethering, or from corporal disproportion. If the penis remains significantly curved after complete takedown of the skin and subcutaneous tissue to the penoscrotal junction, ancillary straightening must be performed. It has been our experience that resection of the urethral plate in the majority of cases will not improve the curvature. We therefore attempt to preserve the urethra plate and correct the curvature by tunica albuginea plications (TAP) a modification of the Nesbit technique. This is performed with permanent sutures (knots are buried) and requires incision through the tunica as described (Page 2560). Note that tunica tissue is not excised. Although some advocate dissecting under the urethral plate to help straighten the penis we have not found this useful and in fact it may be deleterious to the blood supply of the onlay island graft.

5.   A patient with proximal hypospadias undergoes a transverse island tube urethroplasty. After the proximal and meatal anastomosis are complete it is noted that the penis is significantly torsed secondary to tethering from the island flap. Proximal release of the vascularized island tube flap from the penile skin is attempted but the base of the flap is clearly transected and the tube repair looks a bit dusky. What is the next step?

a.   Complete the Byers flap and close.

b.   Remove the dusky neourethra and perform a primary buccal mucosa free graft.

c.   Convert the island tube vascularized graft into a free skin graft by trimming the excess tissue leaving only epidermis and a thin layer of dermis.

d.   Create a proximal meatus to obtain bulky skin coverage and plan for a second stage urethroplasty.

e.   Apply papaverine to the vascularized pedicle graft.

f.   Panic

Correct Answer: c   Reference Page: 2566

Rationale: Once the blood supply to an island flap is violated another choice for urethroplasty must be considered. Free penile skin grafts have been used successfully for both primary and secondary hypospadias. Free grafts require a thin lamina propria so that they may obtain nutrients from the graft bed initially by diffusion followed by new capillary ingrowth. The mistake would be to recognize the injury and not respond by trimming the excess pedicle tissue thereby converting the repair to a free penile skin graft. Using primary buccal mucosa is probably premature for this patient and performing a two stage repair misses the opportunity to use the designed skin since it would have to be discarded or used as a free graft at this point.

6.   **In repairing a fistula after hypospadias surgery a critical consideration is:**

a.   urinary diversion.

b.   mobilization of healthy tissue layers for closure.

c.   repair of associated urethral diverticulum.

d.   identification of other possible fistulas.

e.   confirming the absence of distal urethral stenosis.

Correct Answer: e   Reference Page: 2581

Rationale: All these issues are important in repairing urethral fistulas after hypospadias surgery. However, if urethral stenosis is distal to the stricture, such as meatal stenosis, then an excellent technical repair may fail from high voiding pressures. Urinary diversion is not generally necessary for small fistulas where the repair is performed with healthy tissue using multiple layers. Methylene blue injected into the urethra can aid in identifying other fistulas. Calibrating the urethra with bougie a boules will help identify diverticular fistulas. Injection of saline retrograde via a feeding tube with proximal urethral compression will show ballooning.

7. **After completing a long transverse island tube repair in a case of severe hypospadias you are unable to place a stent into the bladder secondary to a large utricle. The best plan is:**

a. leave the stent out.
b. leave the stent out and place a suprapubic tube.
c. perform endoscopy, pass a wire into the bladder and replace a catheter over the wire.
d. resect the utricle through a perineal incision allowing passage of the catheter
e. stent the repair leaving the catheter distal to the external sphincter and place a suprapubic catheter.

Correct Answer: e   Reference Page: 2554

Rationale: A utriculus masculinus (utricle) is found in ~11% of severe hypospadias cases. The best option is to stent the repair just past the proximal anastomosis and place a suprapubic tube for urinary diversion.

56
Intersex
Bruce Blyth

1. **The genetic material that determines whether a gonad will develop into a testis is carried on the Y chromosome. Which of the following correctly characterizes the gene that provides the signal for differentiation of a gonad into a testis. The gene:**

   a. induces a protein that binds to DNA.
   b. is also known as the H-Y antigen.
   c. is located within the pseudo-autosomal region of the tip of the short arm of the Y chromosome.
   d. codes for a protein that contains a series of zinc fingers.
   e. acts directly to increase transcription.

   Correct Answer: a   Reference Page: 2593
   Rationale: Basic science knowledge of testicular development.

2. **Intersex conditions may arise from mutations and other forms of defective cell division. Non-disjunction is a type of defective chromosomal division that can result in the loss of an X or Y chromosome. Which of the following is correct?**

   a. When non-disjunction results in the loss of an X chromosome, this is noncompatible with life.
   b. Non-disjunction that results in a YO karyotype produces a male phenotype that presents with infertility.
   c. Non-disjunction that occurs after conception is a cause of true hermaphroditism.
   d. Turner's syndrome is a form of non-disjunction with a female phenotype and normal ovaries.

   Correct Answer: c   Reference Page: 2592
   Rationale: Basic science knowledge of types of chromosomal abnormalities producing intersex conditions.

3. **Which of the following correctly describes the development of the gonad into a testis?**

   a.   The gene for testicular development induces the migrating germ cells to enter meiosis.
   b.   The Sertoli cells are the first cells to differentiate in the testis.
   c.   The Leydig cells secrete testosterone, that is a chemotactic factor attracting germ cells from the yolk sac.
   d.   The Sertoli cells differentiate into testicular cords around 80 days of gestation.

   Correct Answer: b   Reference Page: 2594
   Rationale: Basic science knowledge of testicular development.

4. **The development of phenotypic sex is induced by testicular secretions, including androgens and antimullerian hormone (AMH). The following correctly describes AMH:**

   a.   is coded for by a gene on the long arm of chromosome 6.
   b.   is secreted by the Leydig cells of the fetal testis.
   c.   has been shown to enhance the conversion of testosterone to estradiol in the fetal ovary.
   d.   may be defective as a result of a mutation which produces a lethal defect.
   e.   is the first secretion of the fetal testis.

   Correct Answer: e   Reference Page: 2595
   Rationale: Basic science knowledge of testicular development.

5. **The cellular action of testosterone requires binding to the androgen receptor. Which of the following correctly describes these interactions?**

   a.   Testosterone is unable to bind to the androgen receptor.
   b.   The gene for the androgen receptor is carried on chromosome 18.
   c.   The gene for the androgen receptor encodes a protein that contains multiple cysteine residues.
   d.   Androgen receptor abnormalities most commonly result from mutations affecting the concentration of the androgen receptor.

   Correct Answer: c   Reference Page: 2597
   Rationale: Basic science knowledge of testicular development.

6.   **Fertility has been observed in the following intersex conditions:**

   a.   3β-ol-dehydrogenase deficiency, XY karyotype.
   b.   true hermaphroditism.
   c.   mixed gonadal dysgenesis.
   d.   Turner's syndrome.
   e.   Reifenstein's syndrome.

Correct Answer: b   Reference Page: 2601
Rationale: Counseling advice to parents of child with intersex condition.

7.   **The risk of gonadal malignancy is increased in some intersex conditions. In which of the following is the risk of malignancy *not* increased?**

   a.   Mixed gonadal dysgenesis
   b.   Complete androgen insensitivity syndrome
   c.   XY type pure gonadal dysgenesis
   d.   Pseudovaginal perineoscrotal hypospadias
   e.   XX/XY true hermaphroditism

Correct Answer: d   Reference Page: 2601
Rationale: Necessary knowledge for management of intersex conditions.

57

Pediatric Andrology

*Stuart S. Howards, Stanley Kogan, Faruk Hadziselimovic,
Howard M. Snyder, III, Dale Huff*

1.   Peaks in testosterone secretion occur:

a.   at puberty.
b.   randomly before and at puberty.
c.   in the first few months of life and at puberty.
d.   in utero, in the first few months of life, and at puberty.
e.   in utero, in the first few months of life, at 5 to 6 years old, and at puberty.

Correct Answer: e   Reference Page: 2623-2624
Rationale: Before puberty, normal values of LH and testosterone vary with age and one must look up the age-corrected values in order to interpret data from prepubertal children. Figure 57-1 gives the values for LH and testosterone. There is also a spurt in utero. Some experts feel that abnormalities of in utero secretion cause undescended testes.

2.   The incidence of cryptorchidism is:

a.   1% and 66% are unilateral.
b.   1% and 90% are unilateral.
c.   3% and 50% are unilateral.
d.   3% and 66% are unilateral.
e.   3% and 90% are unilateral.

Correct Answer: a   Reference Page: 2629
Rationale: There is some disagreement in the literature regarding the incidence of UDT. One percent is a good approximation, but recent literature suggests that it may be a bit higher. It is useful to share this information with the families because they find it reassuring.

3.   Undescended testis should be repaired at approximately what age?

a.   5 months
b.   10 months
c.   2 years
d.   3 years
e.   4 years

Correct Answer: b   Reference Page: 2629
Rationale: Five months is too young because the testis may descend and there may be increased anesthetic risk. However, most experts recommend early repair. The patients tolerate the surgery better at age 1 than at 2 to 4 years. There also may be a long-term fertility advantage although this has not been absolutely proven.

4.   Infant hydroceles should be repaired at what age?

    a.   5 months
    b.   10 months
    c.   2 years
    d.   3 years
    e.   4 years

Correct Answer: c   Reference Page: 2636
Rationale: Five months is too young because the hydrocele may resolve and there may be increased anesthetic risk. Ten months is also too young because the hydrocele may still resolve although it is not common after 9 to 10 months of age. There is no point in delaying repair beyond the age of 2 years.

5.   Congenital absence of the vas deferens occurs in:

    a.   .01% of males.
    b.   .1% of males.
    c.   1% of males.
    d.   2% of males.
    e.   4% of males.

Correct Answer: c   Reference Page: 2647
Rationale: This is an infrequent, but significant, abnormality. It causes infertility. These patients almost always are carriers of the A gene for cystic fibrosis and should be so advised. The majority are not symptomatic.

6.   Varicoceles in adolescent boys should:

    a.   always be repaired.
    b.   never be repaired.
    c.   be repaired if they are large.
    d.   be repaired if retarded growth of the testis is present.
    e.   be repaired only if the sperm count is low.

Correct Answer: d   Reference Page: 2655
Rationale: There is no consensus as to which varicoceles should be repaired. However, nobody recommends fixing all of them, and most experts do repair them in selected patients. The most common approach is to fix symptomatic lesions or those which have retarded testis growth. Adolescent boys should not be subjected to sperm counts.

7.   **Testes that will not reach the scrotum should be:**

a.   removed.
b.   treated with autotransplant.
c.   treated with staged orchidopexy.
d.   treated by a Fowler-Stephens procedure.
e.   treated by b, c, or d.

Correct Answer: e   Reference Page: 2661-2665
Rationale: The testis should not be removed if it is of reasonable size. All of the listed options are useful depending on the clinical situation and the experience of the surgeon. Transplant is very time consuming and infrequently indicated. Another option is a staged Fowler-Stephens procedure.

58

Pediatric Urologic Oncology

Michael L. Ritchey, Richard J. Andrassy, Panayotis P. Kelalis

1. **A newborn male was noted to have a left renal mass on prenatal ultrasound. Postnatal evaluation confirms a 5 cm solid left renal mass in the lower pole. The right kidney is entirely normal. CXR and CT scan of the chest are negative for metastatic disease. The most likely diagnosis is:**

    a. Wilms' tumor.
    b. intrarenal neuroblastoma.
    c. multilocular cystic nephroma.
    d. congenital mesoblastic nephroma.
    e. renal cell carcinoma.

    Correct Answer: d   Reference Page: 56

    Rationale: In recent years, prenatal diagnosis of many different urologic conditions has been reported. Tumors are no exception. Congenital mesoblastic nephroma is the most common tumor reported in the first six months of life. Although Wilms' tumor has been identified in neonates, it is extremely uncommon. Intrarenal neuroblastoma and renal cell carcinoma are extremely uncommon. Multilocular cystic nephroma would not have the appearance of a solid lesion on ultrasound.

2. **Beckwith-Wiedemann syndrome is characterized by all of the following *except*:**

    a. macroglossia.
    b. hemihypertrophy.
    c. visceromegaly.
    d. Wilms' tumor.
    e. testicular tumor.

    Correct Answer: e   Reference Page: 2684

    Rationale: Beckwith-Wiedemann syndrome is typified by macroglossia and visceromegaly. This includes hepatic enlargement and adrenal cortical cytomegaly. In addition somatic overgrowth is common. Many patients will have hemihypertrophy. Approximately 20% of the patients with Beckwith-Wiedemann syndrome develop malignancies. These include Wilms' tumor, adrenocortical neoplasms and hepatoblastoma.

3.   **All of the following are associated with a decreased survival in patients with Wilms' tumor *except*:**

a.   lymph node involvement.
b.   clear cell sarcoma (CCSK) histology.
c.   rhabdoid tumor of the kidney.
d.   anaplasia.
e.   local tumor spill.

Correct Answer: e   Reference Page: 2682-2683

Rationale: The most important prognostic factors for Wilms' tumor patients are histology and tumor stage. Unfavorable histology patients account for 10% of all Wilms' patients, but account for 50% of deaths. The categories of unfavorable histology include: anaplasia, CCSK and rhabdoid tumor of the kidney. The latter two categories are now not considered to be true Wilms' tumor. Lymph node involvement is one of the most important staging criteria. This is associated with an increased risk of tumor relapse and death. Local tumor spill was found not to have a significant adverse effect on survival. These patients no longer receive abdominal irradiation and have an excellent overall survival.

4.   **Nephrogenic rests have been identified as a precursor lesion of Wilms' tumor. These lesions:**

a.   are found in 20% of kidneys on neonatal autopsies.
b.   are rarely found in bilateral Wilms' tumor.
c.   if present, are associated with an increased risk of development on contralateral Wilms' tumor.
d.   are best diagnosed preoperatively by renal ultrasound.
e.   always develop into Wilms' tumor if left untreated.

Correct Answer: c   Reference Page: 2684

Rationale: Nephrogenic rest is the currently favored term for Wilms' tumor precursor lesions. These were previously termed persistent nodular blastoma, Wilms' tumorlets, or nephroblastomatosis if they were diffuse lesions. Nephrogenic rests are found in 1% of infant autopsies. These lesions are frequently found in patients with bilateral Wilms' tumor and Drash syndrome. These lesions are typically diagnosed by pathologic examination. Although diffuse lesions can be large enough to be seen on imaging studies, this is uncommon. Of the imaging modalities, MRI is most likely to detect these lesions. The majority of nephrogenic rests will involute and only approximately 1 in 80 rests will develop into nephroblastoma.

5. **The following features are associated with favorable prognosis in neuroblastoma:**
a. older age at diagnosis.
b. abdominal location of the primary lesion.
c. metastasis confined to the liver, skin, or bone marrow.
d. n-myc amplification.
e. elevated serum ferritin levels.

Correct Answer: c   Reference Page: 2698-2699

Rationale: Age of diagnosis is an important prognostic factor for patients with neuroblastoma. Survival is inversely correlated with age, with children under age one year performing much better. Thoracic neuroblastoma is associated with a better prognosis than those tumors that arise in the abdomen. There are numerous pathologic criteria and tumor markers that have been employed to stratify patients for treatment. Those with n-myc amplification have a poor prognosis independent of age or stage of disease. Serum ferritin levels are elevated in 50% of the patients with higher stage disease and are associated with a poor prognosis. Stage IV-S patients are those that have metastases confined to the liver, skin, and bone marrow. This is more common in infants and is associated with a favorable prognosis. These patients undergo spontaneous maturation of their tumors.

6. **Teratoma of the testis:**

a. is the most common testicular tumor in children.
b. does not need to be removed as it can be followed with serial tumor markers.
c. regular postoperative chemotherapy to achieve satisfactory survival.
d. follows a clearly benign course in prepubertal children.
e. is typically solid on transcrotal ultrasound.

Correct Answer: d   Reference Page: 2704

Rationale: The most common testicular tumor in children is yolk sac tumor. Teratoma is the second most common testicular tumor of childhood. These tumors typically have multiple cysts which can be identified on ultrasonography leading to the specific diagnosis of teratoma. Prepubertal teratomas have a benign clinical course in distinct contrast to adult cases which have the propensity to metastasize. Those tumors that occur in prepubertal children can be managed with simple orchiectomy. Some centers have advocated testicle sparing procedures as well. Chemotherapy is not necessary.

7. **Which of the following statements is *false* regarding yolk sac testicular tumors in children?**

   a. Most common prepubertal testicular tumor
   b. Characteristic histologic features
   c. Most common site of metastatic spread is to the retroperitoneal lymph nodes
   d. Produces alpha fetoprotein
   e. excellent overall survival exceeding 90%

Correct Answer: c   Reference Page: 2703
Rationale: Yolk sac tumor is the most common prepubertal testicular tumor. A characteristic feature is Schiller-Duval bodies. Cytoplasmic inclusions are common and staining demonstrates the presence of AFP which is typically produced by these tumors. The majority of patients with yolk sac tumor have a good survival which exceeds 95% for all series. Metastases in yolk sac tumors are typically hematogenous. Retroperitoneal lymph node metastases are uncommon. Therefore, retroperitoneal lymph node dissection is no longer routinely used. Imaging studies and tumor markers are relied upon to stage the patient.

8. **Paratesticular rhabdomyosarcoma:**

   a. has a peak presentation between 8 to 10 years of age.
   b. most commonly has alveolar histology.
   c. can be stratified for treatment based on tumor markers.
   d. will spread to retroperitoneal lymph nodes in 28% to 40% of children.
   e. responds poorly to chemotherapy.

Correct Answer: d   Reference Page: 2708-2709
Rationale: The majority of paratesticular rhabdomyosarcomas are of embryonal histology. The peak presentation of these patients is between one and five years of age. Tumor markers have not been identified for this lesion. Retroperitoneal lymph node metastases are common in these patients occurring in 20% to 40% of children. Currently, most children are imaged for the presence of lymph node metastases. Those found to have positive lymph nodes receive chemotherapy. Retroperitoneal lymph node dissection is no longer recommended by the Intergroup Rhabdomyosarcoma Study Group. The majority of patients respond well to chemotherapy. Survival rates have improved from 50% prior to 1970, to the current 90% survival rates.

59
Outpatient Pediatric Urology
Stuart S. Howards

1. **A 12-year-old boy presents with gross hematuria. A complete work-up should include a urinalysis and a(n):**

    a. IVP and a cystoscopy.
    b. sonogram and a cystoscopy.
    c. IVP and work-up for glomerulonephritis.
    d. sonogram and work-up for glomerulonephritis.
    e. IVP, work-up for glomerulonephritis, and 24-hour urine for calcium.

    Correct Answer: e   Reference Page: 2724

    Rationale: Although sonography is now extremely useful and by far more appropriate for most pediatric urologic problems, the patient with hematuria in most settings will benefit from an IVP. This allows one to pick up small calcifications which might be missed by the average sonographer. A cystoscopy is not necessary in these children unless there are persistent symptoms or some complicating factors. They should be evaluated for glomerulonephritis and there is a significant incidence of hypercalciuria in this group of children which can be treated with diuretics in difficult cases although, for the most part, treatment is not indicated. Nevertheless, it is useful to have this information in order to reassure the family.

2. **A 6-year-old girl presents with nocturnal enuresis. She has not had any urinary tract infections and is dry during the day. Her evaluation should include a:**

    a. history and physical examination.
    b. history, physical examination, and sonogram.
    c. history, physical examination, and CMG.
    d. history, physical examination, and VCUG.
    e. history, physical examination, sonogram, and VCUG.

    Correct Answer: a   Reference Page: 2725

    Rationale: Young patients with nocturnal enuresis and no confounding factors do not require any urologic evaluation. If the patient is older and/or the family is very apprehensive, it is reasonable to obtain a sonogram although the yield is extremely low. The sonogram should include an evaluation of bladder wall thickness and a postvoid residual. These will give insight into whether or not there is a neurologic component. However, virtually all children who have neurologic disease also have daytime symptoms and/or urinary tract infections.

3.   **Nocturnal enuresis affects _________ of children 7 years of age and has a spontaneous resolution rate of _________ per year.**

   a.   15%; 20%
   b.   20%; 30%
   c.   7%; 30%
   d.   25%; 10%

Correct Answer: c   Reference Page: 2728

Rationale: Although one can certainly practice excellent medicine without knowing statistics such as the ones called for in this question, it is very helpful and reassuring to the parents if the physician is able to put the problem in perspective. Therefore, it is useful to know the approximately 7% incidence in 7-year-olds and the fact that there is a 15% spontaneous remission each year. This allows them to better make a decision as to whether or not they want to attempt one of the available forms of treatment described later in the chapter.

60
Pediatric Endourology
Gary J. Faerber and David Bloom

1. **A 12-year-old boy has a 6-month history of asymptomatic gross terminal hematuria and postmicturitional bloody spotting. Physical examination is unremarkable. Urinalysis is significant for 5-10 RBC/HPF. The most appropriate step is:**

   a. reassure patient and family that occasional bloody urine in children is normal and no further evaluation is necessary.

   b. intravenous pyelogram or renal ultrasound.

   c. nephrology consult.

   d. upper tract study (intravenous pyelogram or renal ultrasound) and cystoscopy.

   Correct Answer: d   Reference Page: 2739-2740

   Rationale: Gross hematuria in pre-adolescent and adolescent children should be evaluated with an upper tract study and cystoscopy under anesthesia. In a boy this age, cystoscopy under anesthesia would probably be more useful and better tolerated than an awake voiding cystourethrogram. Special attention should be paid to the distal urethra since abnormalities such as dorsal urethral diverticulae, fossa navicularis valves, or urethral polyps have been associated with postmicturition bloody spotting. Miniaturization of endoscopic equipment decreases the risk of traumatic urethral injury.

2. **A 2-year-old boy is undergoing cystoscopy and develops bradycardia and oxygen desaturation. The endoscopist should:**

   a. continue cystoscopy and instruct the anesthesiologist to increase the oxygen concentration and reduce the amount of inhalation agent.

   b. immediately remove the cystoscope.

   c. stop infusion of the irrigant and immediately empty the bladder.

   d. perform cystogram to rule out bladder perforation.

   Correct Answer: c   Reference Page: 2740

   Rationale: Bladder overdistention especially in small children has been associated with cardiac arrhythmias and oxygen desaturation. Immediate drainage of the bladder is oftentimes the only corrective measure needed to correct the problem. The cystoscopist should be cognizant of the amount of irrigant fluid being placed into the bladder.

3.   **The risk of post-operative vesicoureteral reflux is highest after endoscopic incision of ureteroceles of which patient group?**

a.   Neonates with bilateral simple ureteroceles
b.   Older children with large unilateral ureteroceles
c.   Children with duplex intravesical ureteroceles
d.   Neonates with extravesical ureteroceles

Correct Answer: d   Reference Page: 2742
Rationale: Endoscopic incision of extravesical ureteroceles is associated with almost a 50% incidence of post-operative reflux.

4.   **The most common major complication associated with percutaneous nephrostomy in the pediatric age group is:**

a.   urinary extravasation.
b.   tube displacement.
c.   bleeding and sepsis.
d.   hydro/hemothorax.

Correct Answer: c   Reference Page: 2743
Rationale: Major complications associated with percutaneous nephrostomy tubes are 4% which is similar to rates seen in adults. Of particular problem in the pediatric age group is tube displacement; therefore, attention should be placed on securing of the tube.

5.   **The most common complication of pediatric ureteroscopy is:**

a.   urinary tract infection.
b.   vesicoureteral reflux secondary to traumatic dilation of the ureteral orifice.
c.   ureteral perforation.
d.   ureteral stricture formation.

Correct Answer: c   Reference Page: 2743
Rationale: Ureteral perforation is the most common complication associated with pediatric ureteroscopy. The lumen of the ureter is smaller than in the adult ureter and the musculature of the ureter in the pediatric population is less well-developed than in the adult. Therefore, the pediatric ureter is more prone to perforation.

6.	**A 17-year-old girl underwent a continent ileocecocystoplasty using the appendix as the efferent limb. Three years later she developed gross hematuria and abdominal film reveals a 3 x 3 cm calculus in the urinary reservoir. All of the following are reasonable treatment options *except*:**

    a.   direct percutaneous access to the pouch and ultrasonic or electrohydraulic lithotripsy.

    b.   open surgical stone removal.

    c.   flexible endoscopy via the efferent appendiceal limb with electrohydraulic fragmentation and removal of all fragments.

    d.   Dilation of the efferent limb prior to electrohydraulic lithotripsy so that a rigid endoscope can be passed to assist in removal of the fragments.

Correct Answer: d   Reference Page: 2747

Rationale: Open surgical removal of pouch calculi is probably still considered the gold standard for large stones. Smaller stones can be managed endoscopically and removed whole or can be fragmented and removed piecemeal. Access to the pouch via the efferent limb with an instrument too large can damage the continence mechanism. Direct percutaneous access allows for large instruments enabling removal of large pouch calculi.

7.	**A 3-year-old boy has a nonpalpable testis on the right. At diagnostic laparoscopy, spermatic vessels are seen entering to the right inguinal ring. No concomitant hernia is seen on the right. The next step is:**

    a.   terminate laparoscopy, no further intervention.

    b.   right inguinal exploration and contralateral orchidopexy.

    c.   open abdominal exploration for ectopic intraabdominal testis.

    d.   continue laparoscopy to locate the intraabdominal testis and then perform laparoscopic orchiectomy.

    e.   terminate laparoscopy and perform left orchidopexy.

Correct Answer: b   Reference Page: 2749

Rationale: Spermatic cord structures seen entering the inguinal ring indicate that the testis at some point descended at least to the level of the internal ring. Inguinal exploration is warranted because of the relatively high incidence of a gonadal remnant with viable germ cells.